FOOD
AS
MEDICINE
EVERYDAY

FOOD
AS
MEDICINE
EVERYDAY

Reclaim Your Health
With Whole Foods

Julie Briley, ND & Courtney Jackson, ND

NCNM PRESS

Portland, Oregon

Managing Editor: Sandra Snyder, PhD

Illustrations by Jesse Nellis
Photography by Jenny Bowlden and Vanessa Morrow

Published by NCNM Press
National College of Natural Medicine
049 SW Porter Street
Portland, Oregon 97201, USA
www.ncnm.edu

Production: Fourth Lloyd Productions, LLC

Individuals with serious health problems need to be under the care of a physician. Information in this book is intended to supplement, not replace, advice and treatments provided by one's doctor or trained health professional.

Printed in the United States of America

ISBN: 978-0-9771435-6-6 paperback
0-9771435-6-2
Library of Congress Control Number: 2016930290

To FAME series and ECO project participants
—past, current, and future.

Table of Contents

List of Tables

Foreword

My wife, Charlee, and I are in our mid-eighties now, and it seems like only yesterday the people of the world were of average size. The overnight prevalence of obesity and its accompanying ill health seem to have come about rapidly and with great severity in affecting our Western society's health. The public's response to the wholesome whole grain foods we and our company, Bob's Red Mill Natural Foods, have produced over the last forty-one years, brings with it the realization that a nutrient-rich, whole grain diet is one of the key elements to combating the health issues we face today.

Our concern for the world around us—especially children—caused us to look for a vehicle that would address some of these serious health issues. The Ending Childhood Obesity (ECO) project was birthed through our collaboration with the National College of Natural Medicine (NCNM), the naturopathic college in Portland, Oregon. NCNM appeared to be the perfect partnership whereby we could develop a valuable and worthwhile program educating our community about a healthy, whole grain diet, along with an understanding of the basics of good nutritional practices.

NCNM was ready, willing, excited, and they had one very eager physician willing to take on this incredible project: Dr. Courtney Jackson. Within the first year, the popularity of the ECO project was contagious. It soon became necessary to bring on a second physician to help oversee additional classes. Dr. Julie Briley joined the Food as Medicine Institute, and the Food as Medicine Everyday series soon developed following the success of the ECO project. Dr. Briley brought with her the same excitement and commitment to the program. Together they make a dynamite team, educating hundreds of families in the Portland community. They truly are the key to the Food as Medicine Everyday program success.

Charlee and I are so pleased with the growth, continued development, and refinement of the programs coming from the Food as Medicine Institute. Beginning with just one lead naturopathic physician and one twelve-week series, the program has now expanded to five physicians, eighteen series yearly, and has reached over one thousand families to date. This is truly amazing.

At the beginning of our involvement with Dr. Jackson, we talked with her about publishing a book if the project proved successful. We are so pleased to see that the project has proved successful, and here is that book. Congratulations Dr. Jackson and Dr. Briley!

To your good health!

Bob and Charlee Moore

Preface

Food is intimately woven into the culture of naturopathic medical training and clinical practice. Since its inception in the United States in the early 1900s, the profession of naturopathic medicine has always incorporated the healing power of food into patients' prescriptions. The profession has evolved and adapted with modern medicine, but it has not forgotten the original connection to food as medicine. In the United States, naturopathic medicine is currently defined as a distinct system of primary health care that, like conventional medicine, includes the diagnosis, treatment, and prevention of illness. It incorporates the best of both the art and science of traditional and conventional medical practices. NDs are trained to diagnose and treat acute and chronic health conditions, from hay fever to heart disease, from infancy through adulthood. NDs may also provide holistic medical treatment for patients who are using conventional medicine.

Naturopathic medicine is distinguished from other medical professions by its principles:

The Healing Power of Nature (*Vis Medicatrix Naturae*),
Identify and Treat the Causes (*Tolle Causam*),
First Do No Harm (*Primum Non Nocere*),
Doctor as Teacher (*Docere*),
Treat the Whole Person,
Prevention.

This underlying belief in and understanding of the healing power of nature, including the potential for a whole foods diet to prevent, treat, and reverse many chronic diseases, is truly unique to this group of primary care physicians.

When prescribing a treatment plan, naturopathic doctors follow a therapeutic order that does not rely first on prescription medications or surgery. Instead, they may prescribe one of many treatment options to address the whole person. Examples include:

clinical nutrition and prescribing food as medicine

nutritional supplements

botanical medicine

homeopathy

lifestyle counseling

physical medicine, such as soft tissue and joint manipulation

hydrotherapy, the application of hot and cold water to the body to stimulate a
   healing response

intravenous (IV) therapy including vitamin and mineral infusions

minor surgery

prescription medications in some areas of the United States

Naturopathic treatments are in high demand. According to the 2007 National Health Interview Survey, which included a comprehensive survey of the use of complementary health practices by Americans, an estimated 729,000 adults and 237,000 children used a naturopathic treatment in the previous year.[1] Naturopathic doctors also provide something else that patients want from their doctors: time.[2] NDs spend an average of thirty to sixty minutes with their patients, while the average MD may spend seven to fifteen minutes. NDs take time to listen, to understand their patients' concerns and goals, to educate and to create individualized treatment plans.

As a small medical profession, we are stepping up to address the steep rise of chronic diseases in this country that are often based on poor lifestyle choices, including diet. In fact, naturopathic medicine has the potential to fill two significant needs in the current American healthcare system: (1) the lack of access to primary care physicians; (2) insufficient nutrition education provided to conventional medical doctors, preventing them from including appropriate, individualized dietary counseling at each visit.

Within the conventional medical model, a widespread lack of formal nutrition education and clinical application of food as medicine is a known barrier to success in reducing the rates of chronic disease.[3] Compared to conventional medical doctors, NDs are exceptionally well prepared to fill this skill and knowledge gap. NDs complete four required semesters of nutrition training in addition to studies in naturopathic philosophy, which builds a foundation to use food as medicine for mind, body, and spirit. During nutrition courses, NDs receive training in the history, biochemistry, benefits and challenges of prescribing specific diets, such as an anti-inflammatory, low-glycemic, gluten-free, dairy-free, Mediterranean, or vegetarian diet, for example. Additionally, we are trained to utilize diagnostic tests to identify food allergies and food sensitivities and to assess functional digestive problems. Combining this training with extended time face to face with patients, NDs can routinely make a difference in empowering their patients to make dietary changes.

We know that poor dietary choices are one part of the problem of our current healthcare crisis. Food is medicine; therefore, food is part of the solution. It is time that we truly recognize this therapy and that we all learn how to use food as medicine everyday.

Julie Briley, ND
Courtney Jackson, ND

Acknowledgements

To Bob and Charlee Moore, we are honored by your generous support and unwavering encouragement. This book has evolved because of our shared belief in the healing power of whole foods. We value the path we are on together—educating and inspiring families and communities to eat and live well.

Thank you Lori Sobelson, Director of Corporate Outreach at Bob's Red Mill, for your enduring partnership and shared mission to change the way we eat.

We would like to thank David Schleich, PhD, President of National College of Natural Medicine, for his guidance, masterful editing, and for understanding the importance of community outreach in an academic institution.

To Susan Hunter, MBA, Vice President of Advancement at NCNM, for her unrelenting support of naturopathic medicine and the Food As Medicine Institute, and for her counsel from beginning to end.

We were inspired to publish this book because of the life changes we have witnessed over the last several years as a result of our community-based programs. Thank you to all of our Ending Child Obesity (ECO) project and Food As Medicine Everyday (FAME) participants.

We are so grateful to all of the leaders and community members who have supported and helped organize the ECO project and FAME series at the following locations: Mt. Olivet Baptist Church, Schools Uniting Neighborhoods (SUN) Program at Gresham High School and Roosevelt High School, June Key Delta Community Center, White Shield Center, Open Meadows High School and Betties 360, United Methodist Church in Banks, Oregon, Coffee Creek Correctional Facility and NCNM's own Charlee's Kitchen.

A special thanks to Karen and Mark Ward, owners of Jim's Thriftway, for their vision of change in the small town of Banks, Oregon, and to Charlene Zidell for her support of FAME at Coffee Creek Correctional Facility.

We have depended on the dedication and hard work of over one hundred NCNM medical and graduate students to be able to offer programs through the Food As Medicine Institute. The initial student team members in 2010 helped research, develop and design the initial programs and curriculum. Since then, NCNM students continue to be the inspired support staff at workshops every week.

Thank you to Dr. Andy Erlandsen, Dr. Cory Szybala, Dr. Shawnte Yates, our fellow FAMI doctors, for their work and dedication to the FAME series. Our sincere appreciation to Manda Draper, nutritionist and FAMI Coordinator, for her attention to details.

We appreciate the guidance and editing by Nancy Stodart and interior design by Richard Stodart. Thank you to Jesse Nellis, Jenny Bowlden and Vanessa Morrow for bringing this book to life through your beautiful illustrations and photography.

Final appreciation goes to our families for supporting all those weekend *book dates*. Thank you Jeffrey, Maya and Bella. Thank you Doug, Alice and Connor. Writing a book is truly a family affair.

Introduction

When we consider the health report card of Americans, it is no secret that most people have risk factors for chronic diseases such as diabetes, heart disease (still the number one cause of death of Americans), and cancer. These risk factors include a sedentary lifestyle, smoking, drinking too much alcohol, high stress, increased belly fat, and a poor diet. In fact, over 60% of Americans are overweight or obese, which is a significant risk factor for chronic disease.

We are bombarded with messaging, recommendations and guidance from a variety of sources (some reliable, some not) about how we are supposed to make healthy food choices. For example, your doctor tells you to reduce saturated fat and to eat more vegetables. The latest best-seller diet book advises you to increase protein intake, reduce fat, and avoid carbs. Your best friend tells you that by eating certain metabolic-enhancing foods, she finally lost that belly fat, and you can, too!

Most people do indeed want to eat healthier for a variety of reasons: to lose weight; to improve their cholesterol level; to lower blood pressure; or to improve energy. The challenge isn't the desire to eat healthy. The challenge is being able to sift through the varying dietary information sources, understand what is accurate and reliable, and then convert that knowledge into action. For those who have already embarked on improving their diet, initial behavioral changes may have looked something like this: choosing a diet soda over a regular soda; seeking out low-fat labels on food products; declining to add salt to a meal; incorporating *no-calorie* sweeteners, or choosing the latest *low-calorie* breakfast shake. While these examples of changes are made with every good intention for better health, they are often misguided attempts.

The optimal diet we reference throughout this book is based on the Latin word, *diaeta*, meaning *way of living*. We are not referring to a mass-marketed *diet* that promises weight loss and rapid improvements in health. Most such diets are only meant to be followed short-term, as they are too restrictive in their guidelines to be sustainable. Fad diets for sustained weight loss simply don't work by their very definition; they are meant to be short-lived. It has been clearly found that no one diet, whether low-fat or low-carb, is better than another for weight loss.[1] Once you quit a diet, you gain the weight back. This yo-yo effect with weight explains the enormous financial success of the weight loss industry. Fad dieting creates a lifelong weight loss customer.

We also question the guidance of fad diets that, regardless of individual evaluation, encourage people to exclude a complete category of whole foods for improved health, such as grains, meat, or dairy. Not everyone benefits from a diet that is high protein, grain-free, low-fat, or dairy-free. In addition, a vegetarian or vegan diet may be nutritionally risky for some.[2]

This book is not a fad diet book; it is a guidebook that will illuminate the benefits of eating whole foods as a way of living. It will unravel common myths about nutrition so that you can approach food with confidence, not confusion. Physicians, nutrition experts, dieticians, and foodies around the globe are all trying to create the perfect dietary plan for everyone. However, it doesn't exist. There is no single diet that everyone should follow or one that is metabolically correct for all people. Even so, it is important to point out the unifying themes among health-care professionals. Few diets will encourage drinking more soda, eating more white bread, or eating fewer vegetables. We want to showcase what the majority of nutrition experts can all agree upon: eating real, whole foods matters most, and reducing highly processed foods from our diets will lead to better health. This is the way to live for improved health. This is the diet.

There are many contributing factors that influence the likelihood of health or disease in children and adults. One obvious factor is food choice. Simply stated; the Standard American Diet (appropriately nicknamed the SAD diet) is calorie-rich, nutrient-poor, highly processed, and low in whole foods. Poor food choices due to problems of access and education have contributed to our country's epidemic of poor health. As naturopathic doctors, we regularly treat patients dealing with illness and chronic disease due to a lifetime of poor dietary choices. Inspired to expand our work and address community health, we co-founded the Food as Medicine Institute as the National College of Natural Medicine (NCNM). Since 2010, we have facilitated a twelve-week series of community-based nutrition and hands-on cooking workshops called the Ending Childhood Obesity (ECO) project and the Food as Medicine Everyday (FAME) series. We have worked with hundreds of families from diverse cultures and different socioeconomic backgrounds. Time and time again, we observe that participants with widely varied education backgrounds often arrive at the workshops with the same level of minimal nutrition knowledge. They share the same sense of confusion regarding the conflicting and rapidly changing nutrition fads that are widely marketed. Without a solid foundation regarding basic nutrition, it is no wonder that so many of us are swayed to move away from real food. We get easily distracted by all the highly processed, convenient and seemingly cheap products available.

We also understand the obstacles our patients face after they hear dietary advice in their doctor's office and then try to convert that knowledge into real action. People won't eat whole foods if there are obstacles of affordability and availability or if they do not know how to prepare healthy and delicious meals. In our twelve-week cooking and nutrition workshops, we have seen impressive change take place in the lives of participants as they learn to navigate these obstacles in order to develop a healthy relationship with whole food. Far beyond reading a nutrition book or watching a food documentary, we have found it can take at least three months of committed interest and action, such as attending twelve weekly workshops, to empower families and individuals to make sustainable changes in how they spend grocery dollars and cook at home. Our workshops provide multiple opportunities for participants to be in the kitchen with fellow community members. Together they create simple, healthy, and economical recipes. In the end, they realize that they too can purchase and make the same healthy foods at home, and their meals will taste good.

> *Thanks to this group, our family's eating habits have never been better. Each week my family has the opportunity to go and try new foods and cooking styles and learn to eat better. I have become more conscious of the origins of my family's food and of the tremendous varieties that exist right in my own area and to explore new recipes that enrich our diet with locally grown products. This course has been totally wonderful. Our 10-month old son can even eat the food that is made each week, and he LOVES it! I think a LOT of mothers would appreciate how yummy and healthy the classes are.*
> —Christine, ECO project, Mt. Olivet

As you read this book, we hope you will grow confident about making healthy changes to your food choices. To expand this change to have a wider reaching impact on reducing chronic diseases as a nation, especially for our children, we need a family-based, community-based effort. Lack of family involvement in programs aimed at improving children's health and reducing childhood obesity has been identified as the largest barrier to success.[3] The ECO project and the FAME series are bridging this gap in a community-based health revolution.

> There are tons of websites out there focused on health and wellness that you can read, but until you start putting healthy habits into your lifestyle, success cannot be achieved. Dr. Jackson and Dr. Briley educated us on how to incorporate simple practices into our everyday actions through the ECO project. I was thrilled to learn how to make grains and greens that my husband thinks ROCK!

> Since coming to the ECO cooking classes, I look at recipes and how I'm living a bit differently. While I have always been a fit and healthy woman, they inspired me to try new recipes and make some of my already good habits even better! They taught me how to incorporate healthier choices into my busy lifestyle and that it is possible to be a working woman that can provide nourishing fresh meals for her family.
>
> —Jackie, ECO project, Mt. Olivet

If you don't have access to an ECO project or FAME series, don't worry. This book is your beginning. Starting today, you can improve your health and the health of our nation by simply incorporating into your lifestyle sit-down, family dinners made with whole foods.[4,5]

The success we have witnessed by getting individuals and families back in the kitchen, cooking and eating together, inspires us to share what we have seen and learned. This book, or any other nutrition or cookbook for that matter, is no substitute for time spent exploring, preparing and enjoying whole foods. While this book will serve as an excellent nutrition resource, our hope is that it will inspire you to spend time in the kitchen and enjoy a delicious meal.

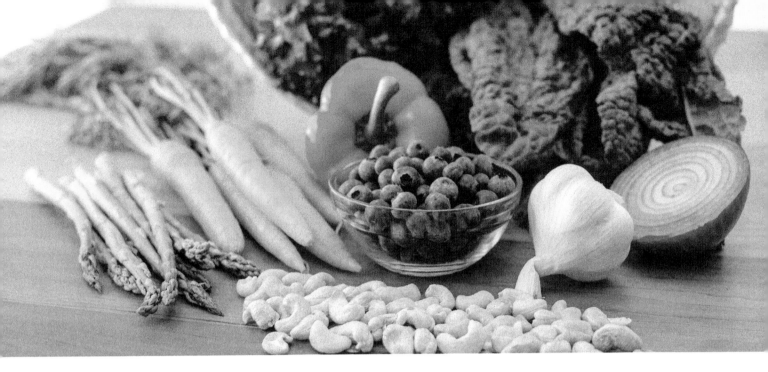

CHAPTER ONE

The Wisdom Of Traditional Diets

If civilized man is to survive, he must somehow incorporate the fundamentals of primitive nutritional wisdom into his modern lifestyle. He must turn his back on the allure of civilized foodstuffs that line his supermarket shelves, and return to the whole, nutrient-dense foods of his ancestors. He must restore the soil to health through nontoxic and biological farming methods. And he must repair that "greatest breakdown in our modern civilized diet", which is the gradual replacement of foods rich in fat-soluble activators with substitutes and imitations compounded of vegetable oils, fillers, stabilizers, and additives.

—Weston A. Price, DDS, *Nutrition and Physical Degeneration*

IN THE DEVELOPED WORLD, WE FIND OURSELVES IN A UNIQUE SITUATION IN THE EVOLUTION OF HUMANKIND. THE GREATEST threat to our well-being is no longer a rival tribe, a feared infectious outbreak, or a large-toothed predator. It is our lifestyle choices that are putting us at great risk.

The United States Centers for Disease Control reports that *non-communicable diseases* (NCDs), such as cancer, heart disease, lung disease, and diabetes are now the major cause of death and disability worldwide. By 2020, NCDs are expected to account for seven out of every ten deaths in the world, as they already do in the U.S. NCDs and the disability, illness, and mortality they cause will soon dominate health care costs.[1] Already, public health officials, governments, and multinational institutions are rethinking how to approach this growing global challenge. According to the World Health Organization, non-communicable diseases are responsible for 63% of deaths worldwide, double the number of deaths from infectious diseases (including HIV/AIDS, tuberculosis, and malaria), maternal and perinatal conditions, and nutritional deficiencies combined.[2] The principal known causes of premature death from NCDs are tobacco use, alcohol consumption, physical inactivity, and poor diet.

Lifestyle choices in the developed world are taking the greatest toll on our health. Rather than letting this grim scenario intimidate you, use this information as the source of a valuable, behavior-changing perspective. We all have a lot of control in mitigating the greatest threat to our health by making changes in daily lifestyle choices. That is something to be excited about!

In this book we will focus primarily on how to move away from the Standard American Diet (SAD), which is highly processed and nutrient-poor, and toward a more whole foods diet. To understand how our current eating habits have brought us to less than ideal health, we must first look back in time.

A Brief History Of Food Production In America

The industrialization of food production in America in the late 1800s included innovations in farming machinery, the building of railroads for food transport, improvements in refrigeration, and the mechanization of food processing. More people were moving into the cities from the country, distancing them from a closer connection to their food. As a consequence for many Americans, there was a shift away from a whole foods, low-processed diet. Ultimately, this transition would contribute to increased rates of chronic disease related to a highly processed diet with decreased nutritional value.

According to the International Food Information Council, 52% of Americans said it is easier to do their income-tax returns than it is to figure out how to eat healthfully!

Grains

Humans began their dietary intake of grains over 100,000 years ago![3] The inclusion of grains in the diet is considered an important part of human evolution because of the complex manipulation required to turn seeds of grain into edible and nutritious food. Wild grains were often dispersed over wide areas, gathered in small amounts by hand, and unavailable certain times of the year. Due to these challenges, grains were eaten rarely and in small amounts.

Our relationship with grains in the diet changed significantly with the domestication of plants about 10,000 years ago. During this agricultural revolution, humans applied lessons learned over tens of thousands of years of grain harvesting and preparation to yield the greatest nutritional benefits from grains year-round. Grains were traditionally prepared by soaking, sprouting, and allowing a natural fermentation to occur for several days before being cooked and eaten. When we study the anatomical parts of a whole grain, we learn that the bran, or outer covering, contains naturally-occurring nutrient inhibitors, such as phytic acid. Phytic acid is the principal storage form of the mineral phosphorus that the plant will ultimately rely upon to grow. Phytic acid is not digestible by humans. Furthermore, phytic acid chelates, or makes un-absorbable, important minerals like zinc, iron, calcium, and magnesium. Generations of humans discovered, through observation, that in order to maximize the nutritional intake of grains in their diet, they needed to cook, soak, ferment, or sprout the grains.[4]

During the Industrial Revolution, planting, harvesting, and processing of grains became faster because of newly invented machinery. In the second half of the 1800s, the number and size of farms increased dramatically, growing commodities such as corn, wheat and cotton. Large scale agriculture in the United States and improved storage allowed for year-round availability of grains to the consumer. Initially, grains were processed via stone milling tools only and retained all their nutritional components: the germ, bran, and endosperm. With the creation of steel roller mills, the germ and the bran were removed, leaving only the endosperm. This starchy part of the grain was then

Phytic acid is not digestible by humans. Furthermore, phytic acid chelates, or makes un-absorbable, important minerals like zinc, iron, calcium and magnesium. Generations of humans discovered, through observation, that in order to maximize the nutritional intake of grains in their diet, they needed to cook, soak, ferment, or sprout the grains.

turned into flour that would not go rancid or spoil as quickly. This processing allowed for the elongation of the shelf life of a food product like white bread or white pasta. Unfortunately, food products made with refined flours have lost valuable nutrition provided by the removed parts. This process of removing parts of the anatomy of the whole grain kernel produces what we now refer to as *refined* grains or flour. Food manufacturers try to compensate for the lost nutrition naturally provided in a whole grain by *enriching* the product with vitamins or minerals.

We've come a long way from hand harvesting wild grains to the daily intake of large amounts of grains in the form of bread, pasta, tortillas, chips, and crackers, all readily and cheaply available to the modern consumer. While some of today's fad diets promote the removal of all grains from the diet due to their refinement and nutrient inhibitors, we promote a return to some of the traditional ways of consuming whole grains; in balanced portions and with proper preparation.

Wild and Cultivated Greens

Like whole grains, wild and cultivated greens have been a part of many traditional diets and are a nutrient-dense food that is often missing from today's Standard American Diet. Dark green leafy vegetables (DGLs) are high in fiber and are a rich source of beta-carotene (the precursor to vitamin A) and vitamin K, both of which are fat-soluble vitamins. Vitamin A is important for vision, immune support, reproduction, and growth. Vitamin K regulates blood clotting and helps maintain mineralization of the bones. DGLs are also a great source of plant-based iron, calcium, and potassium. Traditional diets often prepared greens with a healthy fat source which allowed for increased absorption of these fat-soluble vitamins. An example is cooking collard greens with a ham hock or the traditional use of olive oil with vegetable dishes in the Mediterranean region. Greens are also high in antioxidants, which are important in keeping our bodies from accumulating damaging chemicals, known as free radicals, that contribute to aging and disease.

The process of removing parts of the anatomy of the whole grain kernel produces what we now refer to as refined grains or flour. Food manufacturers try to compensate for the lost nutrition naturally provided in a whole grain by enriching the product with vitamins or minerals.

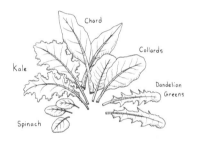

Vitamin A is important for vision, immune support, reproduction, and growth. Vitamin K regulates blood clotting and helps maintain mineralization of the bones. DLGs are also a great source of plant-based iron, calcium, and potassium.

The Standard American Diet is lacking in vegetables, and in particular, dark green leafy veggies. We will introduce several familiar and tasty recipes with greens that will bring this nutritional powerhouse back into your family's diet.

Meat

There has also been a huge shift in meat and poultry production that has increased access in the American diet. Looking at the production and consumption of beef in the U.S., small cattle farms have been replaced by large-scale, industrial meat production. Huge feedlots with cramped conditions for the cattle and large industrial meatpacking plants fueled a massive expansion of cheap, readily available meat.

Small-scale cattle farmers allowed more time for cattle to grow naturally and access to roam and graze on their natural food source, grass. The economics of running a small-scale cattle farm generated a higher cost from this style of raising and slaughtering cattle. Ultimately, this cost was passed on to consumers. Consumers were less likely to purchase high quantities of meat, naturally leading to a more plant-based diet. Meat today is half as expensive as it was in the 1970s.

Small-scale cattle farming was not dependent on growth hormones, which are currently employed in the industrial model to grow fatter cattle, faster. They were also not dependent on antibiotics. Today's meat industry, with its cramped industrial living conditions, is creating sick cattle who often suffer from stomach ulcers due to the unnatural, grain-based diet they are fed. Antibiotic resistance in cattle due to frequent treatment for infections is creating a worldwide problem for humans with the explosion of antibiotic-resistant germs.[5] From a nutritional standpoint, the industrial meat industry is creating less nutritious beef compared to small-scale farmers producing grass-fed beef. Industrial meat contains less vitamin E, beta-carotene, and omega-3 fatty acids.[6] This shift in the essential fatty acid profile of conventional beef makes it prone to contribute to inflammation in the human body.[7,8] In addition, commercially processed meat that makes

Small-scale cattle farming was not dependent on growth hormones, which are currently employed in the industrial model to grow fatter cattle, faster. They were also not dependent on antibiotics. Today's meat industry, with its cramped industrial living conditions, is creating sick cattle who often suffer from stomach ulcers due to the unnatural, grain-based diet they are fed.

its way into hot dogs, lunch meats, and chicken nuggets are high in other additives such as sodium, nitrites and nitrates, and preservatives that can be harmful for the body.

We are concerned that industrial animal agriculture is inhumane and disrespects the natural living and feeding habits of the animals. This model produces less nutritious meat for our consumption and may create new health risks for us because of the drug misuse, unnatural feeding practices, and overcrowding inflicted upon the animals.

Fats

Fat has been considered a highly valuable part of traditional diets. Prior to the establishment of a highly processed food system, populations around the world were sustained and nourished by nutrient-dense, low-processed fats including:

> butter
> beef and lamb tallow
> lard (from pigs)
> chicken, goose, and duck fat
> unrefined coconut and palm oil
> cold pressed extra virgin olive oil
> nuts and seeds
> fish oils, including cod liver oil

Over the last century, the food industry has learned to extract and refine oils from plants like soy, safflower, rapeseed (canola) and corn. They use mechanical and chemical extraction, often bleaching and deodorizing the oils for a neutral color and taste. The Standard American Diet is now high in these processed fats. We have moved away from the days of adding a slab of butter to toast or cooking with lard. But is this wise?

Dr. Westin Price is well known for his 1930's dietary studies of isolated, non-industrialized populations around the world in relation to their dental health. Dental health, including tooth decay and healthy spacing of teeth, can be a window to one's overall health, such as heart health and bone health. Price discovered that these populations had very healthy teeth prior to the introduction of a *civilized diet* that included refined flours and sugar. When refined foods were introduced, good teeth soon deteriorated. Price would ultimately relate these findings, in part, to the natural fat in their diets.

*Price analyzed the primitive diets and found that all contained at least **four times** the quantity of minerals and water-soluble vitamins of the American diet of his day. These diets contained **ten times** the amount of fat-soluble vitamins found in animal fats, including Vitamins A and D. Price considered fat-soluble vitamins to be the key component of healthy diets... Foods that supply vital fat-soluble* *vitamins, as well as other components to aid in their digestion and absorption include butterfat, marine oil, organ meats, fish, eggs, and animal tallows.*[9]

We hear often to eat our greens and veggies. But rarely do we get reminded to eat healthy fats. If we don't eat healthy fat, then we are missing out on a big nutritional opportunity! In Chapter Two, **Nourish Yourself with Fats,** we will discuss how to choose and use healthy fats appropriately to maintain their nutritional value.

FAME Guiding Principles

Following the wisdom of a whole foods diet, our food philosophy will help you learn and make choices about the food you consume. Consider a spectrum of food. On one end is ready-made, highly processed food; on the other end are whole, unprocessed foods. Everyone makes choices somewhere on this food spectrum. Perhaps you are closer to one end, consuming highly processed foods and beverages daily. Or, you may already be committed to a whole foods diet, consuming fresh produce and healthy fats and avoiding processed foods. Most of us fall somewhere in between these nutritional bookends, or even shift back and forth between them. Our goal is to motivate and support choices closer to the whole foods end of this continuum. Rather than jumping from one extreme to the other, this journey is about gradual and sustainable behavior change based on education about food and learning the tools to be successful in your choices. What awaits you is pleasure in the process, enjoying delicious, simple food from recipes we provide. Your relationship with food will change.

The wisdom found in traditional diets and our naturopathic training and clinical experience guided our twelve-week cooking and nutrition courses and this book. The following six guiding principles anchor us as we navigate a whole foods lifestyle in a highly processed food landscape.

- Promote whole foods and low-processed foods.
- Encourage a diverse, primarily plant-based diet.

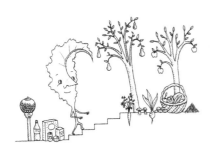

Our goal is to motivate and support choices closer to the whole foods end of this continuum. Rather than jumping from one extreme to the other, this journey is about gradual and sustainable behavior change based on education about food and the tools to be successful in your choices.

- Include food from healthy animals.
- Promote anti-inflammatory food choices.
- Recognize that individuals have unique food needs.
- Care about food and its sources.

Why Choose Whole Foods?

Our post-industrialized society has systematically drifted away from eating whole foods from nature that provide a healthy balance of fat, protein, and carbohydrates. This move away from a nutrient-dense, fiber-rich, whole foods-based diet increases risk of chronic diseases like heart disease and diabetes.

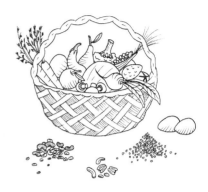

Why Eat a Diverse, Primarily Plant-Based Diet?

Plants like nuts, seeds, whole grains, beans, legumes, fruits and vegetables are nutrient-dense, rich in fiber and antioxidants, and they balance levels of inflammation in the body. On the other hand, a diet based on excess animal products is low in fiber and contributes to increased inflammation in the body. Additionally, meat-based diets are highly resource dependent in an industrial food system in terms of water, feed, antibiotics, and hormones, which puts multiple stresses on the environment.

Why Include Foods from Healthy Animals?

Animals raised in their natural environments produce more nutrient-dense and less inflammatory foods. We encourage a responsible and ethical animal agriculture system that takes into account both the welfare of the animals and the welfare of the environment.

Diets composed of excess added sugar, poor quality fats, conventionally raised meats, and highly processed foods contribute to chronic inflammation. Chronic inflammation affects all systems in the body and contributes to the development of autoimmune, digestive, and neurological disorders, diabetes, and heart disease.

Why Promote Anti-inflammatory Food Choices?

Diets composed of excess added sugar, poor quality fats, conventionally raised meats, and highly processed foods contribute to chronic inflammation. Chronic inflammation affects all systems in the body and contributes to the development of autoimmune, digestive, and neurological disorders, diabetes, and heart disease.

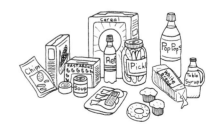

Why Recognize That Individuals Have Unique Food Needs?

There is no one right "diet" for everyone. Life stage, health goals, disease, lifestyle, and food allergies and sensitivities can all influence individual nutritional needs. In addition, individuals' cultural upbringing, food ethics, and access to food must be taken into account regarding dietary recommendations. For example, age determines the need to prioritize certain nutrients over others. Infants require regular intake of fat-rich foods, ideally from breast milk, to support their growing brains. Elders require protein-rich foods to support metabolic changes that may decrease muscle mass. Additionally, specific illnesses ranging from ear infections to diabetes may be prevented or treated by food choices.

Identifying and treating patients with food sensitivities, which is the inability to properly digest certain foods, has been a foundational practice of naturopathic medicine. Food sensitivities or intolerances are common and can be the cause of numerous symptoms, including headaches, mood changes, fatigue, acne, bloating, diarrhea, constipation, menstrual problems, difficulty conceiving, joint pain, rashes, and increased susceptibility to illness. A food sensitivity is the result of an abnormal reaction of the immune system to a food protein. It can be difficult to identify because symptoms may not appear for hours to days after ingesting the food. This differs from a food allergy, which is an immediate response of the immune system that produces an IgE antibody. Food allergies can cause hives, wheezing, swelling and in worst cases, anaphylaxis, a life-threatening emergency.

A person can be sensitive to any food, but the most common foods are soy, corn, dairy, eggs, and wheat—which contains the protein gluten. Dairy sensitivities may be due to a lactase enzyme deficiency called lactose intolerance, or it may be due to an inability to digest one of the milk proteins—casein or whey. Celiac disease differs from (non-celiac) gluten sensitivities, in that it is an autoimmune response triggered by gluten that damages the lining of the small intestine, affecting proper nutrient absorption.

A food sensitivity is the result of an abnormal reaction of the immune system to a food protein. It can be difficult to identify because symptoms may not appear for hours to days after ingesting the food. This differs from a food allergy, which is an immediate response of the immune system that produces an IgE antibody.

Why Care About Food and Its Sources?

Our choice of food can nourish us or it can increase risk for disease. Food connects us to family, community, nature, and the world at large. Food has played a central role in the social interaction of humans for thousands of years. We must begin to understand the connection between food production and food choice and how it relates to health, happy humans, and a healthy environment.

Macronutrients—The Big Players of Nutrition

A diverse whole foods-based diet provides a complete range of nutrition components that is often absent in a highly processed diet. This includes healthy sources of fat, carbohydrates rich in fiber, and protein. Let us review some basics about nutrition which can help you better understand and communicate the value of whole foods. To begin, we will look at the importance of macronutrients.

Macronutrients are nutrients required in large amounts for a healthy body: fats, carbohydrates, proteins, and water. All of these nutrients are needed by the body because they provide energy, function, and structure. For instance, the brain needs all three macronutrients because it is composed of fat and protein and requires glucose (a carbohydrate) to function. Water is required by every system in the body. In the next three chapters, we focus on the importance of healthy carbohydrates, protein, and fats in the diet.

"

I came into the FAME series not understanding whole foods. I have learned so much about nutrition that I thought I knew, but didn't.

I am more creative in the kitchen converting recipes to healthier choices. I have found my family has learned through my healthier choices and we are growing as a family in a healthy way. I have lost over 22 pounds in the 12 weeks.

—Sherry, FAME Series,
　Charlee's Kitchen

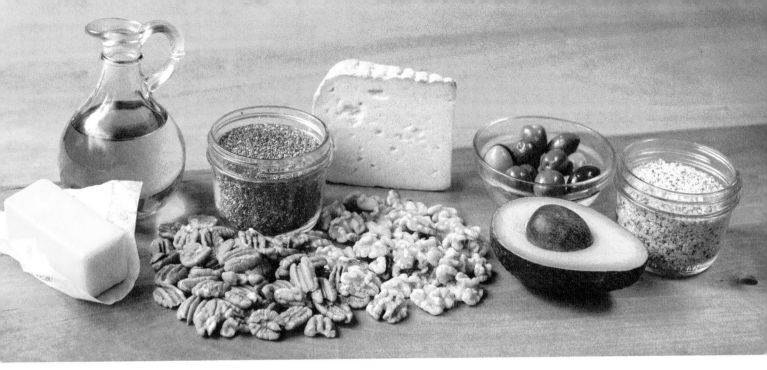

CHAPTER TWO

Nourish Yourself With Fat

Eat Healthy Fat. It's Good For You!

THE SUBJECT OF FAT IN OUR DIET IS CONTROVERSIAL. IN THE LAST FEW DECADES, AMERICANS HAVE HEARD CONFLICTING messages about whether to eat a low-fat diet, a diet rich in unsaturated fats, or a diet low in saturated fats. Every year the information dispensed to the public is changing. We aim to demystify some of the confusion about fat in our diet because *healthy fat is good for us*. Unfortunately, many Standard American Diet eaters are hesitant to include healthy fat on their plate.

Let's begin with a few basics to clarify some of the confusion about healthy fat before diving deeper into our fat discussion:

- Fats are an essential nutrient to include in a daily diet. Healthy fat can include both saturated and unsaturated fats found in both plant and animal whole food sources.

- The best fats to include are those that are less processed and remain closer to their natural form.

- Smoking or overheating oils when cooking will cause oxidation to the fat, thereby increasing the risk of harm to the body. Polyunsaturated fats are at greater risk of becoming oxidized compared to saturated fats due to the differences in their chemical structure.

- Cholesterol is a type of fat naturally produced by your liver as well as a type of dietary fat. Food sources of cholesterol come from animal foods such as eggs, meat, and dairy. Much misguided information has been promoted about the role of cholesterol and disease. Cholesterol-rich foods can, in fact, be a part of a healthy diet.

- Every person has individual nutritional needs including which fats to include in the diet.

Nutrition Language Of Fats

Understanding the nutrition language of fats will help us to navigate the conflicting messages we have heard and help us to communicate clearly about the different types of fats in food, including saturated, unsaturated and trans fats.

To begin, fat is an energy-dense nutrient providing nine calories per gram compared to four calories per gram from protein and carbohydrates. The body digests fat more slowly than proteins or carbohydrates. Fat in your food can give you long-term energy, or what we like to call *slow fuel*, for the day, and helps to give you a satiated feeling from a meal. Fat surrounds and protects all the cells in your body, and the fat you eat is incorporated into those cell membranes. This is why it is essential to choose healthy fats and to avoid dangerous trans fat, which we will discuss soon. Dietary fat helps the body to absorb essential fat-soluble vitamins, which are vitamins A, D, E, and K. Natural sources of fat in the diet come from both plants and animals and may include items in Table 2.1.

A quick review of some basic biochemistry is needed to understand the difference between saturated and unsaturated fat. The chemical structure of fat has a glycerol base with three fatty acid chains attached. It is the fatty acids that can be saturated or unsaturated, which is a chemistry reference to how many double bonds occur within the fatty acid chain. Saturated fat contains no double bonds. Unsaturated fat contains one or more double bonds. The number of double bonds influences the physical characteristics of the fat. For instance, oils rich in unsaturated fat, like olive, flax, avocado, or sesame, tend to be liquid at room temperature. Compare these to saturated fats, like butter, lard, or coconut oil, which are solid at room temperature.

Table 2.1 Food Sources of Fats

Animal Sources Of Fats	Plant Sources Of Fats
Dairy: butter, milk, cheese and yogurt (full-fat) Egg yolk Fish Meat, poultry, and animal skin	Avocado Cocoa/chocolate Coconut Nuts and seeds Olives and olive oil

SOURCES OF
MONOUNSATURATED FATS

> Olives and olive oil
> Avocados
> Peanuts
> Sesame seeds
> Chicken Fat
> Lard

SOURCES OF POLYUNSATURATED FATS

High in omega-3 fatty acids

> Fish (salmon, trout, halibut,
> cod, sardines)
> Pasture-raised meats
> Flaxseed *
> Chia seed *
> Walnuts *

High in omega-6 fatty acids

> Corn oil
> Soybean oil
> Safflower oil
> Conventionally raised meats

_____

*High in omega-3 fatty acid precursors.

Unsaturated Fats

The body relies on unsaturated fat to create and balance a healthy level of inflammation. Additionally, unsaturated fat surrounds and protects nerve cells, including those of the brain and eyes. Unsaturated fat includes both monounsaturated and polyunsaturated fat. The mono (one) and poly (many) refer to the number of double bonds within the fatty acids. The number of double bonds in a fat influences the way it reacts to heat, light, and oxygen in the environment, a process called oxidation. The oxidation of the fat creates unhealthy free radicals and eventually causes the oil to become rancid. Polyunsaturated fats are less stable than monounsaturated fats when exposed to oxygen, or higher heat, because they have multiple double bonds. Overheating plant-based polyunsaturated fats from soy, canola, sunflower, or corn oil is associated with atherosclerosis and inflammatory joint disease.[1] Unfortunately, many highly processed, packaged foods tend to contain these exact oils, increasing our exposure to oxidized fats.

Polyunsaturated fats are also referred to as essential fatty acids because the body doesn't naturally make them. These include omega-3 and omega-6 fatty acids. The key is to choose quality fats and to avoid an excess of highly processed omega-6-rich oils.

The Balancing Act of Omega-6:Omega-3

Americans are consuming polyunsaturated fats, omega-3 and omega-6, out of balance. In general, most omega-3 fatty acids tend to reduce inflammation in the body while omega-6 fatty acids tend to promote inflammation. A healthy ratio of omega-6 to omega-3 in the diet ranges from 4:1 to 6:1. Americans are now often eating a 16:1 to 20:1 ratio, leading to health consequences associated with increased inflammation.[12] Omega-3 fatty acids are found in most fish (salmon, tuna, sardines, cod), and nuts and seeds (walnuts, flax, chia). Higher levels of omega-6's are found in oils from corn, soybean, safflower, and sunflower, which are often cheaper, highly-processed oils. Omega-6 oils are frequently used in creating packaged and fast foods because they are inexpensive for food manufacturers to include. One can see how the Standard American Diet has contributed to this imbalanced ratio. To improve this ratio and to promote an anti-inflammatory diet, we recommend reducing your intake of omega-6 fatty acids from highly processed oils, namely corn and soybean, which are often called vegetable oil. In addition, increase the amount of omega-3 fatty acids-rich foods in the diet as another important way to improve this ratio.

Saturated Fats

Saturated fats surround and protect your brain as well as provide energy for your heart. They support cell membranes, providing necessary stiffness and integrity, and assists in the absorption of fat-soluble vitamins like A, D, E, and K. High consumption of poor quality saturated fat (from conventially-raised animal products) along with low intake of fiber and antioxidants from fruits and vegetables is linked to inflammation, high cholesterol, and heart disease.[2] Eating saturated fat in balance with unsaturated fat as part of a whole foods diet is healthy. Saturated fats are provided in the diet by both animals and plants. Because saturated fat is more chemically stable, it is a good choice to cook with at higher temperatures.

Trans Fat: A Fat to Avoid

You've heard our message: Eat healthy fat. It's good for the body. However, there is one type of fat to avoid: trans fat.

ANIMAL SOURCES OF SATURATED FATS

Dairy products (whole milk, cheese, butter)
Bacon, sausage, and processed meats
Poultry skin (duck, chicken, turkey)
Fatty cuts of meat
Egg yolks

PLANT SOURCES OF SATURATED FATS

Coconut oil
Chocolate
Palm oil

*All major medical governing bodies, including the American Heart Association and the American Diabetes Association, agree that **trans fats should be completely avoided** in the diet because of the strong link to heart disease and unhealthy changes in the brain.*

SOURCES OF TRANS FATS

Margarine
Shortening
French fries and most fried foods
Packaged baked goods

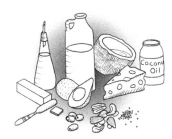

Scientists have discovered that bombarding unsaturated fats with hydrogen atoms creates trans fats, a far cry from a low-processed, natural fat. Another name for trans fat is *partially hydrogenated oils*.

Trans fat is created to give food a longer shelf life: it goes rancid less quickly. This fat is often used in the fast food industry for frying and for stabilizing packaged food products. Another motivation to use trans fat by industrial food producers is their bottom line. They use cheaper, low quality oils that are at risk for oxidation to create these trans fats. This is turn provides a cheaper food product for the consumer, although at a cost to your health.

Trans fat increases inflammation in the body and is linked to heart disease and Alzheimer's disease.[3,4] All major medical governing bodies, including the American Heart Association and the American Diabetes Association, agree that **trans fats should be completely avoided** in the diet because of the strong link to heart disease and unhealthy changes in the brain.[5] Chapter Five, **Reading Food Labels**, will help identify possible sources of trans fat in food.

Demystifying Dietary Fat

Now that we know the different types of dietary fat available to us, let's dive into the fat conflict. Media and health professionals present conflicting messages about *good* and *bad* fats, often solely promoting the health benefits of unsaturated fats and the health consequences of saturated fats. Additionally, cholesterol in food is often villainized. This misguided, overly simplistic advice about Good Fat/Bad Fat can be traced back to the work of researcher Ansel Keys in the 1950s and 1960s. The data he collected influenced United States Department of Agriculture (USDA) food policy recommendations for a low-fat diet for decades to follow.

Mr. Keys conducted what is referred to as the *Seven Countries* study. From data collected, Mr. Keys reported high dietary intake of fat contributed to high cholesterol levels which increased rates of cardiovascular disease. One of the controversies surrounding Mr. Keys' findings is that prior to this study, he had access to additional dietary and health data from over twenty countries, and the complete data showed that *some countries exhibiting high dietary fat intake also displayed lower heart disease levels*. Little attention was given to following up with those countries reporting high-fat diets and low heart disease levels.

With conflicting information about the role of dietary fat, cholesterol, and heart disease, it is troubling to consider why the USDA presented one overly simplistic point of view to the American public for the last few decades. Heart disease is STILL the number one cause of death for both men and women in this country, and *no-fat* or low-fat dietary advice for the masses has not led us as a nation to better health outcomes.

Interestingly, excess dietary carbohydrates stimulate the body to produce the types of saturated fats known to inhibit proper cardiovascular functioning. Take note: excess refined and simple carbs from soft drinks and potato chips actually create a greater health risk associated with blood levels of saturated fat than healthy sources and portions of naturally fatty meat, butter, and cheese made from healthy animals.[6]

Demystifying Cholesterol

Cholesterol continues to be a subject on the receiving end of much name-calling in the health and food industry. So what exactly is cholesterol and why do we care so much about it? Cholesterol is a type of fat made by the body and also consumed in the diet. Cholesterol forms the building blocks of sex hormones—including estrogen, progesterone, testosterone, DHEA—and vitamin D. It supports the structure of all the cells in the body, including brain cells. Cholesterol helps to repair damaged tissue in the body due to its role in creating healthy cell membranes. The liver makes 75% of your total cholesterol levels, leaving only 25% to be influenced by dietary intake. The liver takes care of regulating the body's need for cholesterol in response to internal metabolic influences.[7] Some of the metabolic triggers that can lead to an elevated cholesterol level may include

Cholesterol continues to be a subject on the receiving end of much name-calling in the health and food industry. So what exactly is cholesterol and why do we care so much about it? Cholesterol is a type of fat made by the body and also consumed in the diet. Cholesterol forms the building blocks of sex hormones—including estrogen, progesterone, testosterone, DHEA—and vitamin D.

low thyroid function, diabetes, stress and other diseases associated with the stress hormone cortisol, as well as genetic tendencies. As for dietary intake, the body is built to regulate liver cholesterol production in relation to increased or decreased dietary intake of cholesterol.

We have all heard of *bad* cholesterol, aka low-density lipoprotein or LDL, especially in relation to its colleague, high-density lipoprotein or HDL, known as the *good* cholesterol. Most Americans are concerned about elevated cholesterol and heart health. A lot of current dietary advice is aimed at "lowering total cholesterol" levels because of the association of elevated cholesterol with heart disease and heart attacks. This is another area that needs demystification. *An elevated total cholesterol level, as measured through a lab test, does not predict your chance of having a heart attack.* Indeed, a 2009 national study analyzing over 135,000 Americans showed that nearly 75% of patients hospitalized for a heart attack had cholesterol levels that would indicate they were not at high risk for a cardiovascular event by current conventional standards.[8] The physiology of cholesterol in the body is more complex than the simple name-calling of *Good HDL* and *Bad LDL* that you may hear in most doctors' offices. There are different types and sizes of both HDL and LDL that have shown different impacts on the development of heart disease. Rarely do doctors do the deeper study of analyzing the various sub-types of HDL and LDL.

Assessing one's cholesterol level continues to be part of the standard of care for determining heart disease risk. However, the development of heart disease is a multifaceted process and includes significant and equally important factors besides total cholesterol and dietary intake of fat. This includes hypertension, tobacco use (smoking or chewing), physical inactivity, obesity, diabetes, poverty, chronic stress, depression, and excessive alcohol intake. Risk factors that you do not have control over include a family history of heart disease, male gender, advancing age, and African ethnicity. If you do have many risk factors for heart disease or if you have established heart disease, then the following choices can be a healthy response:

The physiology of cholesterol in the body is more complex than the simple name-calling of Good HDL and Bad LDL that you may hear in most doctors' offices. There are different types and sizes of both HDL and LDL that have shown different impacts on the development of heart disease. Rarely do doctors do the deeper study of analyzing the various sub-types of HDL and LDL.

reducing your consumption of poor quality saturated fat and refined carbohydrates, improving the quality of your dietary fat, and working to lower elevated total and LDL cholesterol level and triglycerides. These choices must be paired with many other lifestyle modifications to address other risk factors listed above. On the flip side, having too low a cholesterol level can lead to its own health concerns, such as an inability to produce sufficient sex hormones as well as to mental health diseases, such as depression.[9]

In our work teaching community nutrition and cooking classes, we hear from many participants who are avoiding whole eggs or egg yolk to avoid the cholesterol, due to concern about the relationship between high cholesterol and heart disease. Eating cholesterol in the diet (yes, even from eggs) above the recommended USDA guidelines of 300 mg has been shown to raise both the protective large HDL and the large LDL.[10] So, unless you have an egg allergy, an egg intolerance, or you have been identified as someone whose cholesterol specifically reacts to eggs, which is a small minority of people, eat those eggs, preferably made from healthy, pasture-raised chickens.

To bring this complex topic to a close, *The International Journal of Clinical Practice* has cleared up this Good Cholesterol/Bad Cholesterol debate with this statement: "The earlier purported adverse relationship between dietary cholesterol and heart disease risk was likely largely over-exaggerated."[11] When conflicting research presents itself, it is always a good idea to return to what we know for a fact about the way the human body works. *Human physiology dictates that we must have adequate cholesterol in the body for good health.*

If you have been told you have elevated cholesterol, we recommend you do the following: work with a naturopathic doctor who is trained to understand the physiology of cholesterol in the body and who can appropriately guide you based on the total amounts, the particle types, and the balance of your cholesterol levels in relation to your overall health.

Unless you have an egg allergy, an egg intolerance, or you have been identified as someone whose cholesterol specifically reacts to eggs, which is a small minority of people, eat those eggs, preferably made from healthy, pasture-raised chickens.

Bringing Fat Back To The Kitchen

Recall that we mentioned the nutrient-rich, low-processed fats, including butter, tallow, lard, coconut and olive oil, that have nourished populations around the world. Knowing how to properly cook with fats is just as important as choosing low-processed fats; recall the negative health implications of overheating polyunsaturated fat, including increased risk of inflammatory diseases. Certain fats withstand higher heat, like most saturated fats and certain unsaturated fats with higher smoke points. The reality is that some degree of oxidation will occur with cooking oils. Eating antioxidant-rich foods is very important to counteract the negative health effects of any oxidized fats in the diet. Antioxidant-rich foods include brightly colored fruit and vegetables, beverages such as tea and coffee, and dark chocolate.

You will find that in many of the recipes included in this book (see **Recipes**), we recommend using low-processed, natural fats. This includes coconut oil, avocado oil, butter, or animal fats for higher heat needs, such as baking and sautéing, and extra virgin olive oil for recipes that require lower temperature cooking, as well as for salad or meal dressings. Unrefined expeller pressed sesame oil can be used for its distinctive flavor in stir-fries, sauces, and dressings. It generally has a medium-to-high smoke point. Avocados and walnuts are naturally high in healthy fats, thus requiring less processing to extract the oils, but they can be more expensive at the grocery store. Grapeseed oil, which can be a sustainable by-product of wine production, is often marketed for its neutral flavor and may be an economical choice at the store. However, the seeds have very high amounts of omega-6 fatty acids (about 70%) and often undergo extensive processing, increasing the risk of oxidation. With any oil you choose, be sure to review the oil's smoke point and avoid overheating the oil. Refer to Table 15.4 and Table 15.5 in Chapter Fifteen, **Kitchen Skills**.

The topic of whether canola oil is a healthy choice is a common question in our workshops. Canola oil is often marketed as having high omega-3 content. It is important to look beyond marketing and consider the source and production of this particular oil.

You will find that in many of the recipes included in this book (see **Recipes***), we recommend using low-processed, natural fats. This includes coconut oil, avocado oil, butter, or animal fats for higher heat needs, such as baking and sautéing, and extra virgin olive oil for recipes that require lower temperature cooking, as well as for salad or meal dressings.*

Canola oil comes from the rapeseed plant, which is an inedible plant in its natural form because it contains a toxic compound, erucic acid. Originally, rapeseed oil was used for lamp fuel and as an industrial lubricant. In the early 1970s, the plant was bred to contain a lower amount of its toxic compound, leading to the name: **Ca**nola or **Ca**nadian **O**il **L**ow **A**cid. To extract the oil from the tiny rapeseeds, a high amount of processing must occur. This includes chemical extraction (using hexane, a petroleum-based product), high heat, and bleaching, exposing the sensitive omega-3 oils to stressors that contribute to the oxidation of the fatty acids.[13,14] The very thing that canola oil is marketed for, the high omega-3 content, is compromised.

In addition, the rapeseed plant is recognized as one of the most common genetically modified organisms, or GMOs. Learn more about why we encourage limiting or avoiding GMOs in food products in Chapter Five, **Reading Food Labels**. Increasing omega-3 fatty acids in the diet is a healthy goal. However, we do not support the use of canola oil. There are more natural and less processed fats that will increase omega-3 fatty acids in the diet, including ground flaxseed, chia seed, walnuts, egg yolks from pasture-raised chickens, grass-fed beef, and many types of fish.

And Finally—The Question Everyone Is Asking— Does Eating Fat Make You Fat?

Get ready for this... No. Eating healthy, low-processed fat is good for you and your waistline.[15,16] When avoiding all fat in the diet, people tend to eat more simple carbohydrates to feel full, which can definitely contribute to weight gain. In 1977, public health recommendations for the U.S. population were made to reduce fat intake to less than 30%. Food producers responded to this recommendation by replacing fat with carbohydrates. We have since learned that contrary to those recommendations, replacing dietary fat, specifically saturated fat, with carbohydrates likely increases the risk of heart disease. Additionally, increased carbs cause an increase in blood glucose, which

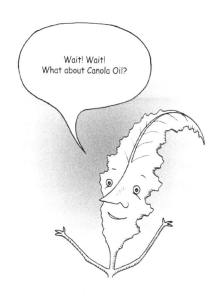

Wait! Wait! What about Canola Oil?

Originally, rapeseed oil was used for fuel lamps and as an industrial lubricant. In the early 1970s, the plant was bred to contain a lower amount of its toxic compound, leading to the name: Canola or Canadian Oil Low Acid.

stimulates the hormone insulin and promotes fat cell growth around the midsection. Avoiding fat in the diet does not lead to a smaller waistline, and quite frankly, your food doesn't taste as good.[17]

Read a label on a *fat-free* or low-fat product and see what has been added to compensate for the loss of flavor from the fat; often it is sugar and/or salt. Remember, fat provides slow fuel for your day and helps you feel satiated. We will teach you the balancing act of building a healthy plate that contains healthy fat as well as carbs and protein.

The bottom line: you can learn to optimize the quality and quantity of fats you cook with and eat to support a healthy metabolism.

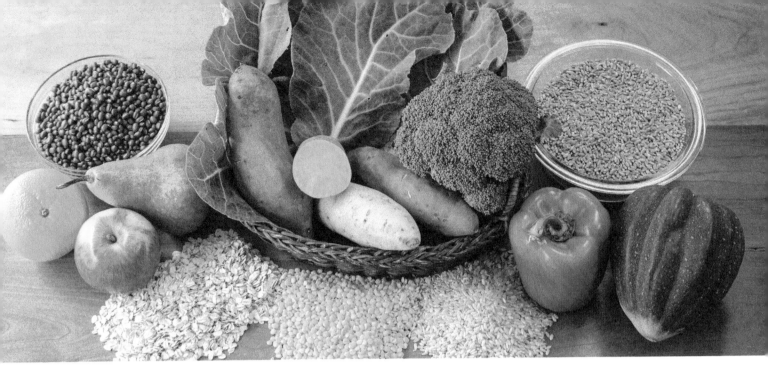

CHAPTER THREE

Nourish Yourself With Carbohydrates

IF THERE IS A MACRONUTRIENT CATEGORY THAT AMERICANS ARE FAMILIAR WITH, IT'S CARBOHYDRATES! WE LOVE OUR CARBS. Consider the last time you consumed pasta, bread, cereal, chips, popcorn, rice, fruit juice, soda pop, beer, wine, or an energy drink. These foods and food products are jam-packed with carbohydrates, some healthier than others. While many are highly processed, there are whole food sources of carbohydrates, including some of our favorites: green leafy kale, carrots, sweet potatoes, black beans, brown rice, and whole fruit. Plant foods will provide the large majority of carbohydrates in our diet.

Carbohydrates serve numerous benefits in our body, including:

energy for the brain from glucose,
fuel storage in the form of glycogen,
food sources of phytonutrients, which are plant-based chemicals that support health, including anti-oxidants from fruits and veggies,
satiety, balanced cholesterol and regulation of bowel movements from fiber.

It is important to navigate carbohydrates well: choosing poorly can lead to weight gain, insulin resistance, cavities, heart disease, increased inflammation, and decreased immune function.

Learning the language of carbohydrates is important before venturing into label reading. Starches, fiber and sugar all refer to carbohydrates.

Carbohydrates exist in two main categories: complex and simple. Complex carbs are longer chains of simple carbs and are also called polysaccharides (many sugars). They provide slow energy compared to simple carbs. Simple carbs come in two sizes and may be referred to as monosaccharides (or single sugar) or disaccharides (two sugars).

Here are common sugar chains that make up carbohydrates:

SIMPLE CARBOHYDRATES

Simple carbohydrates generally taste sweet and provide quick energy. Eaten in excess and without a balance of fats and protein, they can lead to blood sugar spikes and crashes. Excessive sugar intake is also associated with weight gain, poor dental health, and diabetes.

Monosaccharides

Glucose: Main source of energy for the brain

Galactose: Creates lactose or milk sugar

Fructose: Sweetest of all sugars, found in fruit and honey

Disaccharides

Sucrose or table sugar (glucose + fructose)

Lactose or milk sugar (glucose + galactose)

COMPLEX CARBOHYDRATES

Complex carbs provide a slower fuel for the body due to the longer time needed to digest and the feeling of fullness provided by the fiber. Polysaccharides are *many chains* of sugars; they form food sources of fiber and starch.

Fiber is a complex carbohydrate that is indigestible, but has many benefits.

Starch is a complex carbohydrate that can be digested and broken down into simple sugars.

Table 3.1 Food Sources of Simple and Complex Carbohydrates

Complex Carbohydrates	Simple Carbohydrates

Legumes and beans
Nuts and seeds
Vegetables
Whole fruits
Whole grains
	Sugar
	Fruit juice
	Sweetened beverages:
	  soda, tea, energy drinks
	Honey, maple syrup, agave
	  nectar
	Refined grains:
	white pasta, white bread

Their Effects In The Body	**Their Effects In The Body**
Provide slow energy for your body and brain Fiber helps the body remove waste and excess cholesterol Increase the sense of fullness after eating Provide important fuel to sustain friendly bacteria in the gut	Provide quick energy for your body and brain Taste sweet Excess can lead to cavities, weight gain, and diabetes

Let Fiber Be Your Guide

Fiber is a powerful guide in your journey towards a more plant-based diet. Excellent food sources of fiber include: whole fruits; vegetables; beans, peas, and other legumes; nuts and seeds; and whole grains. Notice that plant foods provide fiber (through their cellulose content) while animal products, such as meat and dairy, do not. The fiber content of whole foods is compromised when it is highly processed, such as, whole fruit into fruit juice, vegetables into vegetable juice, and whole grains into refined grains.

While starches are complex carbohydrates that break down into sugar, fiber is an indigestible complex carbohydrate which has numerous benefits. Fiber is categorized as *soluble* or *insoluble*. Soluble means the fiber attracts water, which creates *bulk* in your gut, slows down digestion, and contributes to a sense of fullness. Sources of soluble fiber include: apples, pears, oatmeal, beans and lentils, nuts, flaxseeds and psyllium. Insoluble fiber, on the other hand, remains relatively unchanged in your gut and contributes to regular bowel movements, preventing constipation. Sources of insoluble fiber include whole grains, nuts and seeds, and dark green leafy vegetables. *Both* types of fiber can be found in many plants and *both* are important to include in the diet.

Normalizing bowel movements is one of the many benefits of fiber. It helps to bulk up and soften the stool, making for an easier passage. Increase your fiber intake slowly making sure to support increased fiber with adequate hydration. Fiber and water work well together to relieve constipation and maintain healthy bowel elimination. Don't be surprised if you experience increased gas with more fiber. As your intestines adjust to their new environment, the gas will diminish. A high-fiber diet supports long-term colon health.[1]

Fiber also helps to maintain healthy cholesterol levels by assisting the removal of cholesterol from the body through bile secretion.[2] Soluble fiber found in beans, oats, and flaxseed helps lower total cholesterol levels and supports a heart-healthy lifestyle by reducing risk factors associated with heart disease.[3,4]

Another benefit is that fiber helps control blood sugar levels. Soluble fiber, for example, slows the absorption of dietary sugars in the digestive tract, which can help balance blood glucose levels. A diet that includes *insoluble* fiber has also been associated with a reduced risk of developing Type II diabetes.[5,6,7] A high-fiber diet can also aid in weight loss and the reduction of belly fat.[8,9] Obesity and increased belly fat are two risk factors for heart disease and diabetes. Increasing dietary fiber is a simple strategy to reduce risk of these common conditions.

High-fiber foods will provide a sense of fullness and satiety with meals, decreasing the likelihood of overeating and unnecessary snacking. Generally speaking, high-fiber foods found in whole vegetables

Fiber is categorized as **soluble** *or* **insoluble**. *Soluble means the fiber attracts water, which creates* bulk *in your gut, slows down digestion, and contributes to a sense of fullness. Insoluble fiber, on the other hand, remains relatively unchanged in your gut and contributes to regular movement of the bowels, preventing constipation.*

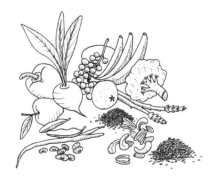

and whole fruits tend to be lower in calories per serving. A telling example of this is drinking one cup of apple juice (approximately 115 calories, 0 grams of fiber, 24 grams of sugar) compared to eating one whole apple with the skin on (approximately 65 calories, 3 grams of fiber, 13 grams of sugar). In addition, the sugar in the juice now contributes to *added sugar* in the diet, which we will discuss in depth in Chapter Eight, **Exploring Sweeteners.**

Whole Grains

Whole grains can be a delicious source of high-fiber foods in any meal. Examples of whole grains include: barley, brown rice, buckwheat, millet, oats, whole corn, whole wheat, wild rice, quinoa, teff, and amaranth. We previously discussed the change in processing of whole grains over time; let's now take a closer look at the change in nutrition, including fiber content, when whole grains are refined.

Whole grains provide complex nutrition from the combination of all of its parts, including the bran, germ, and endosperm.

The **bran** is the outer protective layer of the grain, (also refered to as the husk or shell) which protects it from germinating until it is in the optimal environment. Not only is it a protective fibrous layer for the grain, it is an excellent souce of dietary fiber. It also provides B-vitamins and trace minerals like iron. B-vitamins are an important part of many biochemical processes to create energy in the body and support a healthy nervous system. Iron is required in red blood cells for proper oxygen transport.

The bran also contains an anti-nutrient called phytic acid, which prevents the plant from germinating in less than ideal environments, but for humans, can *prevent* the absorption of minerals, such as calcium, magnesium, iron, and zinc. Certain cooking methods such as soaking, sprouting, and fermenting can decrease the amount of phytic acid and other nutrient inhibitors in whole grains.

The germ is the part of the grain that contains the genetic information for the plant to germinate or initiate growth. It provides essential fatty acids (a combination of omega-3 and omega-6) as well

B-vitamins are an important part of many biochemical processes to create energy in the body and support a healthy nervous system. Iron is required in red blood cells for proper oxygen transport.

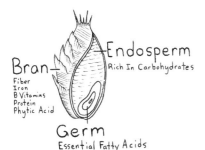

Bran
Fiber
Iron
B Vitamins
Protein
Phytic Acid

Endosperm
Rich In Carbohydrates

Germ
Essential Fatty Acids
Protein
Vitamin E
B Vitamins
Iron

as vitamin E. The vitamin E, an antioxidant, works synergistically with the essential fatty acids, to protect these valuable oils from oxidation. It is *natural* for real food to spoil over time. Thus, food manufacturers remove this whole grain part to ensure a longer shelf life, which robs us of this valuable combination of nutrients.

The **endosperm** contains the necessary energy (carbs and protein) for a seedling to initiate growth. It consists of starch, a digestible complex carbohydrate that the body breaks down into simple sugars. It also contains protein and some B-vitamins. Refined grains are the result of processing out the germ and the bran, leaving only the starch-rich endosperm.

So, how much fiber do you need? Our Paleo ancestors are thought to have consumed over 100 grams of fiber a day! Today, the average American male consumes 16 to 18 grams a day, and females 12 to 14 grams a day.[10] Naturopathic doctors generally recommend 35 to 50 grams a day of fiber intake as a realistic and important goal. Aiming to increase the amount of fiber up to 50 grams daily will naturally propel you toward a whole foods, plant-based diet.

So, in the end, what's not to love about fiber?

A couple of simple ways to increase fiber in your diet is to eat a whole piece of fruit and skip the juice or to choose whole grains (brown rice, for example) over refined grains (white rice). Add vegetables to every plate. Include fiber-rich foods alongside foods that contain no fiber: meat, dairy, poultry, and eggs. Beans and legumes can provide a fiber-rich alternative to animal protein at some meals. Refer to the chart to see how you measure up with your daily fiber intake.

Naturopathic doctors generally recommend 35 to 50 grams a day of fiber intake as a realistic and important goal. Aiming to increase the amount of fiber up to 50 grams daily will naturally propel you toward a whole foods, plant-based diet.

Table 3.2 Food Sources of Fiber

Fresh & Dried Fruit	Serving Size	Fiber (g)
Apple with skin	1 medium	5.0
Apricot	3 medium	1.0
Apricots, dried	4 pieces	3.0
Banana	1 medium	4.0
Blueberries	1 cup	4.0
Cantaloupe, cubes	1 cup	1.0
Figs, dried	2 medium	3.5
Grapefruit	½ medium	3.0
Orange	1 medium	3.5
Peach	1 medium	2.0
Pear	1 medium	5.0
Plum	1 medium	1.0
Raisins	1.5 ounces	1.5
Raspberries	1 cup	6.5
Strawberries	1 cup	4.5

Grains, Beans, Nuts & Seeds	Serving Size	Fiber (g)
Almonds	¼ cup	4.0
Amaranth, cooked	1 cup	5.0
Black beans, cooked	1 cup	14.0
Bread, whole wheat	1 slice	2.0
Brown rice, cooked	1 cup	4.0
Cashews	¼ cup	1.0
Chia seed, dry	2 tablespoons	10.0

Table 3.2 Food Sources of Fiber (cont'd)

Grains, Beans, Nuts & Seeds	Serving Size	Fiber (g)
Corn, sweet	1 cup	4.5
Flaxseed, ground	2 tablespoons	4.0
Garbanzo beans, cooked	1 cup	6.0
Kidney beans, cooked	1 cup	11.5
Lentils, red, cooked	1 cup	13.5
Lima beans, cooked	1 cup	8.5
Oats, rolled, cooked	1 cup	5.0
Quinoa, cooked	1 cup	8.5
Pasta, whole wheat	1 cup	6.0
Peanuts	¼ cup	2.0
Peas, cooked	1 cup	9.0
Pistachio nuts	¼ cup	3.0
Popcorn, air-popped	3 cups	3.5
Pumpkin seeds	¼ cup	4.0
Sunflower seeds	¼ cup	3.0
Walnuts	¼ cup	3.0

Vegetables	Serving Size	Fiber (g)
Avocado (fruit)	1 medium	12.0
Beets, cooked	1 cup	3.0
Beet greens	1 cup	4.0
Bok choy, cooked	1 cup	3.0
Broccoli, cooked	1 cup	4.5
Brussels sprouts, cooked	1 cup	3.5

Table 3.2 Food Sources of Fiber (cont'd)

Vegetables	Serving Size	Fiber (g)
Cabbage, cooked	1 cup	4.0
Carrot, raw	1 medium	2.5
Carrot, cooked	1 cup	5.0
Cauliflower, cooked	1 cup	3.5
Collard greens, cooked	1 cup	2.5
Green beans	1 cup	4.0
Celery	1 stalk	1.0
Kale, cooked	1 cup	7.0
Onions, raw	1 cup	3.0
Peppers, sweet	1 cup	2.5
Potato, baked with skin	1 medium	5.0
Spinach, cooked	1 cup	4.5
Sweet potato, cooked	1 medium	5.0
Swiss chard, cooked	1 cup	3.5
Tomato (fruit)	1 medium	1.0
Winter squash, cooked	1 cup	6.0
Zucchini, cooked	1 cup	2.5

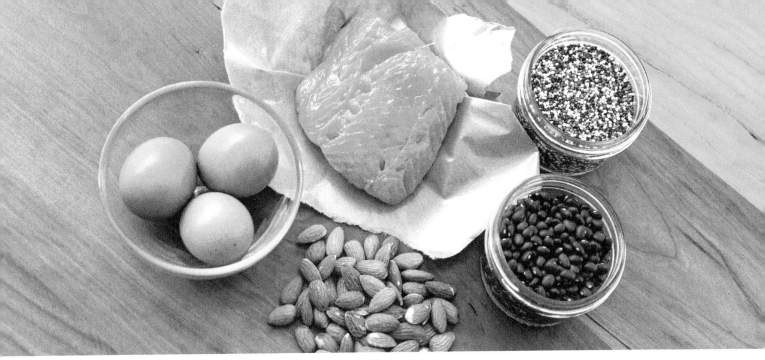

CHAPTER FOUR

Nourish Yourself With Protein

PROTEIN IS AN ESSENTIAL MACRONUTRIENT COMPOSED OF BUILDING BLOCKS CALLED AMINO ACIDS. PROTEIN PROVIDES STRUCTURE in the body in the form of connective tissue, bone, hair, and muscle. It creates the framework of antibodies in the immune system, of hormones like insulin and gastrin in the digestive system, and of neurotransmitters in the brain. Protein, through the formation of enzymes, controls *every chemical reaction in the body*. From a dietary perspective, protein serves as a slow fuel energy source, along with fat and complex carbohydrates.

Animal sources of protein include beef, pork, lamb, buffalo, wild game (venison, elk), poultry, fish, eggs, and dairy foods such as milk, cheese, and yogurt. Plant-based protein sources include nuts like almonds, pistachios, and walnuts; seeds like hemp, chia, sunflower, and pumpkin; all beans and legumes; and whole grains.

A diet low in protein, or a diet based on poor quality protein, contributes to many symptoms such as fatigue, mood instability, difficulty building muscle, lackluster hair, and hormone imbalance.

There are nine amino acids that human bodies must acquire through the diet in order to create proteins. These are called *essential amino acids* and include:

histidine
isoleucine
leucine
lysine
methionine
phenylalanine
threonine
tryptophan
valine

Nonessential amino acids are made by the body from essential amino acids or through other metabolic processes in the body. They include:

alanine
asparagine
aspartic acid
glutamic acid

The body may require an increase of certain *conditional* amino acids during times of illness and stress. These include:

arginine
cysteine
glutamine
glycine
ornithine
proline
serine
tyrosine

The importance of consuming adequate amino acids—and therefore protein—cannot be understated in terms of its impact on a healthy body and a healthy mind. Recall the various roles of protein

The importance of consuming adequate amino acids—and therefore protein—cannot be understated in terms of its impact on a healthy body and a healthy mind.

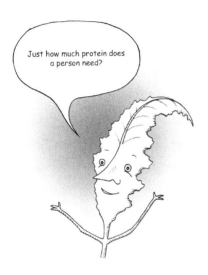

Just how much protein does a person need?

Determining an individual's protein requirements can be complicated because the amount needed changes with age, health status, pregnancy and breastfeeding, activity level and fitness goals. In addition, digestive capacity and metabolism can influence the use of dietary protein. The generally accepted recommendation is 0.8 grams per kilogram of body weight for adults.

in the body that include supporting the physical structure of the body as well as hormone and neurotransmitter production. In certain situations, naturopathic doctors will expand upon a food-based recommendation and prescribe individualized amino acid therapy in order to support specific chemical pathways in the body. For instance:

- **Tryptophan** converts into serotonin and melatonin, both of which support a healthy mood and restorative sleep.
- **Tyrosine** converts into stress hormones like adrenaline as well as thyroid hormone.
- **Phenylalanine** converts into pain-relieving endorphins.
- **Glutamine** provides a fuel source for the brain and enterocytes, cells that line the small intestine.
- **Arginine** converts into nitric oxide, a potent chemical that relaxes blood vessels.
- **Cysteine** supports the creation of one of the body's most potent antioxidants, glutathione.

Determining an individual's protein requirement can be complicated because the amount needed changes with age, health status, pregnancy and breastfeeding, activity level, and fitness goals. In addition, digestive capacity and metabolism can influence the intake of dietary protein. The generally accepted recommendation is 0.8 grams per kilogram of body weight for adults. This translates to:

a 150-pound person (equal to 68 kg) consuming approximately 55 grams daily.

a 200-pound person (equal to 91 kg) consuming approximately 73 grams daily.

Another way to think about an individual's protein requirement is by calculating a percentage of daily caloric intake. The Institute of Health's *Dietary Reference Intake* (DRI) and the USDA recommend anywhere from 10% to 35% of total calories to come from protein for normal, healthy adults. For example, eating a 2,000 calorie diet, one could consume anywhere from 50 grams (that's 10% of calories) to 175 grams (35%) of protein per day.

A low-glycemic index diet, which encourages a lower intake of carbohydrates and higher intake of fats and proteins, recommends 20% of daily caloric intake to come from protein. In a 2,000 calorie diet, this equals about 100 grams.

With such a wide range of potential protein intake, it can be beneficial to seek individualized advice. A naturopathic doctor can assess your individualized dietary needs relating to metabolic health, healthcare goals, and medical concerns and determine a healthy range of protein intake. For those with a history of kidney disease, it is essential to get guidance on protein intake, because excess protein can place stress on the kidneys.

Check Table 4.1 to compare different food sources of protein. Be sure to compare animal sources with plant sources. Look for foods that are rich in protein compared to foods that would require consuming a large quantity to meet a general guideline of daily protein intake between 60 to 100 grams. Notice that animal foods (including meat and dairy) are excellent sources of protein, followed by legumes and seeds.

A low-glycemic index diet, which encourages a lower intake of carbohydrates and higher intake of fats and proteins, recommends 20% of daily caloric intake to come from protein. In a 2,000 calorie diet, this equals about 100 grams.

Table 4.1 Food Sources of Protein

Animal Food	Serving	Protein (g)
BEEF	3 ounces	21
CHICKEN	3 ounces	25
PORK	3 ounces	19
FISH	3 ounces	21
EGGS	1 large	7
DAIRY		
Milk	1 cup	8
Yogurt	1 cup	8 to 12
Cottage cheese	½ cup	15
Hard cheese	1 ounce	7

Plant Food	Serving	Protein (g)
BEANS (black, pinto, lentils)	½ cup cooked	7 to 10
NUTS and SEEDS		
Almond butter	2 tablespoons	8
Peanut butter	2 tablespoons	8
Almonds	¼ cup	8
Peanuts	¼ cup	8
Pecans	¼ cup	2.5
Cashews	¼ cup	5
Sunflower seeds	¼ cup	6
Pumpkin seeds	¼ cup	8
Ground Flaxseed	2 tablespoons	4

Table 4.1 Food Sources of Protein (cont'd)

Plant Food	Serving	Protein (g)
VEGETABLES		
Broccoli	1 cup	5
Cauliflower	1 cup	3
Spinach	1 cup	3
Carrots	1 cup	1
Asparagus	6 spears	1
FRUIT		
Avocado	1 large	4
Dates	1 cup	4
Raisins	1 cup	4
Orange	1 medium	2
Banana	1 medium	1

Good Things Come in Small Packages—The Role of Micronutrients

Now that we have detailed the macronutrients (fat, carbohydrate, and protein) and emphasized the need to include all three in a healthy diet, we will focus on the smaller, but still important micronutrients. Vitamins and minerals are micronutrients that occur in very small quantities in food. Vitamins occur mostly in plant and animal sources, while minerals can be found in plant, animals, water, and soil. By eating a whole foods-based diet, you will naturally introduce rich sources of vitamins and minerals into your body. Highly processed foods often have these important nutrients removed or altered from their natural state. Check Table 4.2 and Table 4.3 to learn basic functions and whole food sources of these micronutrients.

Table 4.2 Vitamins: Functions and Food Sources

Vitamin	Functions	Food Sources
A (Vitamin A Palmitate, Beta-carotene)	Supports eyes and enhances immunity Antioxidant Fat-soluble*	Orange, yellow, and dark green vegetables (carrots, squash, spinach, kale), liver, pasture-raised beef, egg yolks, and poultry
The Bs (Thiamin-B1, Riboflavin-B2, Niacin-B3, Pantothenic acid-B5, Pyridoxine-B6, Biotin, Cobalamin-B12, Folate-B9)	Supports numerous chemical reactions in the body that impact mood, energy, neurological development, and detoxification	Dark green leafy vegetables, meat, poultry, eggs, whole grains (bran), nutritional yeast
C (Ascorbic acid)	Supports immunity, collagen production, energy production, and blood vessels	Broccoli, cauliflower, citrus fruit, peppers, berries, melons
D (Cholecalciferol-D3, Ergocalciferol-D2)	Supports immunity, bone health, growth, and mood Fat-soluble*	Fish (specifically cod liver oil), milk from pasture-raised cattle and goats, mushrooms, *and sunshine—the best non-food source*
E (Tocopherols)	Antioxidant Fat-soluble*	Whole grains (germ), nuts and seeds, dark green leafy vegetables
K (Phylloquinones-K1, Menaquinones-K2)	Supports blood clotting and bone health Fat-soluble *	K1-Dark green leafy vegetables K2-Produced by friendly gut bacteria

* Fat-soluble indicates that dietary fat is needed to absorb the vitamin.

Table 4.3 Minerals: Functions and Food Sources

Minerals	Functions	Sources
Sodium	Keeps fluid in balance in the body and supports energy Excess amounts may affect blood pressure in some people	Salt, processed and canned foods, seaweed
Potassium	Supports nerves, heart, muscles, and stress tolerance	Avocado, kiwis, bananas, cantaloupe, melons, spinach and other dark green leafy veggies
Calcium	Builds strong bones and teeth	Dark green leafy vegetables (kale, spinach, broccoli), almonds, fish and animal bones, dairy, sesame seeds
Iron	Binds and transports oxygen in the blood	Red meat, dark green leafy vegetables, molasses
Magnesium	Regulates blood pressure, smooth muscle relaxation and healthy stress response	Vegetables (especially dark green leafy veggies), nuts, seeds, beans
Zinc	Immune support, wound healing and healthy mood	Red meat, eggs, oysters, pumpkin seeds

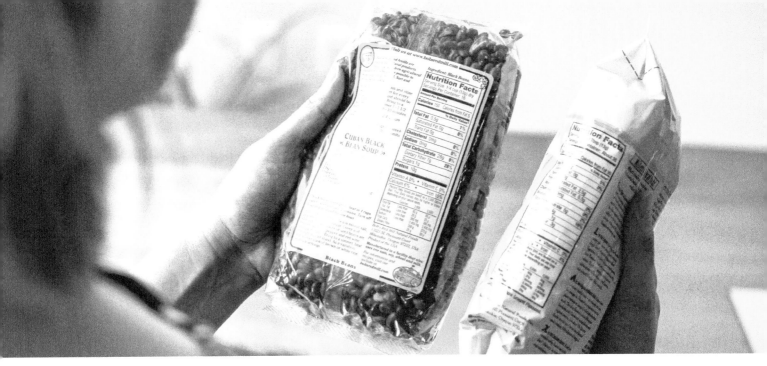

CHAPTER FIVE

Reading Food Labels

I used to go shopping and buy groceries without looking at labels. Now, I look at all the labels on all items. I looked at a bottle of lemonade, and it had 26 grams of sugar per serving. I learned that a female's daily intake of "added" sugar should be no more than 24 grams. So, I had to walk quickly away from the lemonade.

—Beryl, ECO project, Mt. Olivet

I could really connect with the idea of moving towards whole foods. This idea helped in choosing foods at the grocery store (reading food labels and buying organic from the Clean 15 list) to eliminating foods containing additives, chemicals, and sugar. The changes affect my whole family. Thank you!

—Kathy, FAME series, Charlee's Kitchen

IN ORDER TO MAKE THE HEALTHIEST CHOICES POSSIBLE WHEN SHOPPING, SKILLS AND CONFIDENCE IN READING FOOD LABELS ARE important. When initially reading a label, many people will first look at the numbers and percentages in the Nutrition Facts section regarding the amount of fat, calories, sodium, or cholesterol. Other consumers may initially be attracted to the health claims on the front of the food label, such as low-fat, *heart-healthy*, or *all natural*. Food claims on the front of food packaging may have little to do with the actual nutrition in a food. Rarely does the conventional food industry have your health first and foremost in mind, and they will often use manipulative language on labels to sway your shopping habits.

Food label reading is an acquired skill that initially requires practice. Our goal is to provide guiding priniples to follow as you begin this important habit. A bit of extra time at the grocery store dedicated to reading food labels will be time well spent. It will not be a perfect process, but it can be empowering as you choose the foods and ingredients you will be consuming and thereby impacting your health and the health of your family. Even small changes can have a huge impact on health.

Getting Started Reading Food Labels

You may find that the following food items either do not have a food label or only have one ingredient listed on the label: fruits, vegetables, fresh meats, poultry, fish, bulk nuts, seeds, legumes, and whole grains. A single listed ingredient often indicates a whole food that has not been processed. However, when purchasing boxed, canned, and prepared food, you will be confronted with more complex labels. Taking time to compare the labels of similar products can have a great impact on your health once you learn to recognize ingredients and misleading label claims. Oftentimes there are convenient and more nutritious alternatives to highly processed foods containing less additives, refined grains, and sugars.

Most shoppers are familiar with locating the two basic parts of a food label: **Nutrition Facts** and **Ingredients**. As we work to promote the benefits of a whole foods diet, we are going to reprioritize the process of food label reading and encourage you to begin at one particular spot: the Ingredients. *Let the Ingredients section of the label be your initial guide to a whole foods lifestyle.*

Steps For Reading A Food Label (Refer To Label 1)

Step 1: The Ingredients

This is the best place to start for understanding what is in the food and the level of processing that may have taken place. Assess the following, in order:

Length of the List: Without even reading the ingredients, take a look at the length of the list. The number of ingredients in a product can give you an idea of the degree of processing and the amount of additives. In general, when a product contains a large number of ingredients, it is likely that it contains additives such as preservatives, food coloring, and added flavors.

Ingredients: Everything on the list should be a recognizable food item. If it is not, it is likely a highly processed food or a chemical additive. Next time you are shopping, ask yourself what you would expect to find in the food product if you were making the same thing at home. For example, if you are making a pot of

Popular Canned Chili

INGREDIENTS: Water, Beef, Cereal (oatmeal, corn flour), Chili Powder, Textured Vegetable Protein (soy flour, caramel color), Tomatoes (water, tomato paste), Sugar, Salt, Hydrolyzed Corn Protein, Hydrolyzed Wheat Protein, Modified Food Starch, Flavors, Autolyzed Yeast, Monosodium Glutamate, Spices.

Label 1

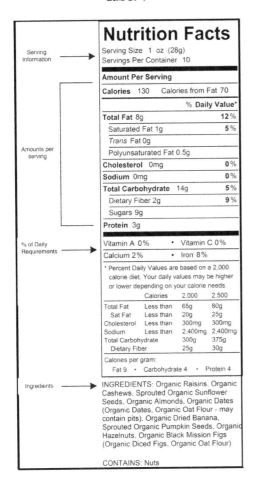

chili at home, you might add beans, tomatoes, spices, onions, garlic, and other vegetables. Then, look at the ingredient list of a canned chili and compare what is common and what is surprising with a homemade version. Would you expect to find texturized vegetable protein, monosodium glutamate (MSG), oatmeal, modified cornstarch, or autolyzed yeast in your chili? Probably not!

Order of the ingredients: The ingredients are listed in order of the greatest amount to the least amount. Thus, the order will give you a good idea of what the main ingredients are in a food product.

Within the ingredients list, pay special attention to:

> *added sweeteners*
>
> *sugars*
>
> *fats*
>
> *refined grains*
>
> *chemical additives*

Added Sweeteners and Sugars

Some foods may contain more than one type of sweetener, such as evaporated cane juice, brown rice syrup, corn syrup and molasses, for example. (Label 2) Each sweetener is added to the food in smaller quantities, which allows it to be individually listed further down on the ingredient list. However, if you were to combine all the added sweeteners, it may likely be the highest quantity ingredient in the product. Food companies can employ this tactic as a way to avoid having to list *sugar* as the number one ingredient. Also, foods that claim to have *no sugar*, may have added artificial sweeteners instead. We will discuss these highly processed sweeteners in a later section, but these are chemicals that should be avoided in a whole foods diet.

Label 2 represents a breakfast cereal and lists the food's

second ingredient as marshmallows, which contain three types of sweeteners: sugar, dextrose, and corn syrup. In addition, further down on the label, two more sweeteners are listed: sugar and corn syrup. This results in 10 grams of refined sugars per serving, which is equivalent to 2½ teaspoons of sugar in a ¾ cup serving! Considering that most people would eat two servings (1½ cups) or more of this cereal in a sitting, this equates to 20 grams or 5 added teaspoons of refined sugar. This is dangerously close to the daily maximum amount of added sugar for most adults (more to come on this topic) and not a great way to start the day.

Fats

Read the ingredient list for any fats or oils that have been *partially hydrogenated*; this term signifies that the product has trans fats. The trans fats most likely to be encountered on a food label are partially hydrogenated soybean oil and partially hydrogenated cottonseed oil. If a product contains fully *hydrogenated oils*, it does not mean it is a trans fat. It does signify a very highly processed fat and should ideally be avoided. The trans fats we refer to are the highly processed partially hydrogenated oils added in food to increase their shelf life. In 2015, the FDA approved changes that will require the removal of added partially hydrogenated oils from processed foods due to their negative health effects. However, food producers have several years to implement these changes, so continue to read food labels carefully.

Read Label 3 and notice that the Nutrition Facts breakdown of Total Fat lists Trans Fat at 0 grams. But, upon reading the ingredient list, you will find *partially hydrogenated lard*, which IS a trans fat!

Label 2

Nutrition Facts

Serving Size   3/4 Cup (27g)
Servings Per Container   About 16

Amount Per Serving		
Calories 260	Calories from Fat 20	
		% Daily Value*
Total Fat 1g		2%
Saturated Fat 0g		0%
Trans Fat 0g		0%
Polyunsaturated Fat 0g		0%
Monounsaturated Fat 0g		0%
Cholesterol 0mg		0%
Sodium 170mg		7%
Potassium 50mg		1%
Total Carbohydrate 22g		7%
Dietary Fiber 2g		6%
Sugars 10g		
Other Carbohydrate 10g		
Protein 2g		3%
Vitamin A 10%	•	Vitamin C 10%
Calcium 10%	•	Iron 25%
Phosphorus 4%	•	Magnesium 4%

INGREDIENTS: Whole Grain Oats, Marshmallows (sugar, modified corn starch, corn syrup, dextrose, gelatin, calcium carbonate, yellows 5&6, blue 1, red 40 (artificial flavor), **Sugar, Oat Flour, Corn Syrup, Corn Starch, Salt, Trisodium Phosphate, Color Added, Natural and Artificial Flavor, Vitamin E** (mixed tocopherals) **added to preserve freshness.**

Important Information On Trans Fats

There can be up to 0.5 grams of trans fats per serving in a food product before it is required to be noted in the Nutritional Facts portion of the label. Remember to look at the Ingredients section of the label for the type of oil used and not to rely on the claim that a product has 0 grams of trans fats on the front of the label or in the Nutrition Facts, as that may be completely false.

Label 3

Nutrition Facts

Serving Size   1/4 Cup (38g/1.3 oz.)
Servings Per Container   About 6

Amount Per Serving

Calories 170   Calories from Fat   50

	% Daily Value*
Total Fat 4.5g	7%
Saturated Fat 2g	9%
Trans Fat 0g	0%
Polyunsaturated Fat 1g	0%
Monounsaturated Fat 1g	0%
Cholesterol <5mg	1%
Sodium 340mg	14%
Total Carbohydrate 27g	9%
Dietary Fiber <1g	2%
Sugars 7g	
Protein 2g	

Vitamin A 0%	•	Vitamin C 0%
Calcium 8%	•	Iron 6%

INGREDIENTS: WHEAT FLOUR, DEGERMINATED YELLOW CORN MEAL, SUGAR, ANIMAL SHORTENING (CONTAINS ONE OR MORE OF THE FOLLOWING: LARD, HYDROGENATED LARD, PARTIALLY HYDROGENATED LARD), CONTAINS LESS THAN 2% OF EACH OF THE FOLLOWING: BAKING SODA, SODIUM ACID PYROPHOSPHATE, SALT, MONOCALCIUM PHOSPHATE,

Remember—trans fats in the diet contribute to unhealthy changes in cholesterol levels, increased inflammation in blood vessels, and negative effects in the brain.[1,2] Even a small amount in the diet can have these negative effects. Avoiding trans fats completely is the healthiest option. Unfortunately, many people may be consuming more trans fats than they realize if they are not checking food labels and reading the ingredient list. This is especially true of consumers of packaged and processed foods such as margarine, baked goods, and fried or frozen meals.

Refined Grains

A food may be marketed as being a *whole grain* product even if it has mostly refined grains and only a small portion of whole grains. A common example is *Whole Wheat Bread*. Check out the number one ingredient listed: often it will be refined wheat flour. Avoid this marketing trap by looking for products that list *100% whole grains* on the label. Remember to confirm any claims on the front of the label with what is actually in the ingredient list. When reading a food label for grains and flours, the following are examples of whole grain ingredients: whole wheat, brown rice, whole corn or cornmeal, and whole oats. The following words signify that it is not a whole grain: refined, white, enriched, and degerminated.

Chemical Additives

Chemicals may be added to a food item to enhance its color, flavor, or shelf life. While the FDA has claimed many of these additives to be *Generally Recognized as Safe*, most food additives have not actually been tested to rule out long term health consequences associated with regular intake in adults or children. We recommend avoiding or limiting any chemical additives in foods to reduce any individual reactions and to decrease the body's need to process and eliminate chemicals. Chemical additives can have wide-ranging negative effects such as: allergies, asthma, headaches, joint pain, hyperactivity, foggy thinking, dizziness, chest pain, depression and mood swings, fatigue, weight gain, diarrhea and other digestive complaints.[3,4,5,6]

The most common additives to avoid and their food sources are listed below. Again, the only place to find this information is in the **Ingredients**.

Artificial Colors: Look for these listed as a color and a number, for example, yellow #5 or red #40.

Artificial Sweeteners: Aspartame (Nutrasweet® and Equal®), sucralose (Splenda®), saccharin (Sweet N Low®), and acesulfame potassium are the most commonly used artificial sweeteners.

Preservatives: Added to many meats, boxed and canned foods to lengthen shelf life, here are some examples of common preservatives:

Sodium nitrites/nitrates are typically found in processed deli meat, sausages, and hot dogs.

Sulfites are often added to dried fruits and wine.

BHS, BHT and EDTA can be found in canned goods.

MSG (monosodium glutamate): A flavor enhancer once added to many processed foods, it is still used in some popular snack food brands, soups, and salad dressings.

Olestra (an artificial fat): This was a popular additive used in the 1990s when the low-fat craze was in full swing. Its most common effect is acute diarrhea, for which it fell out of popularity. Unfortunately, you can still find it in popular brands of *light* potato chips.

Certain food additives that enhance flavor are actually known in the science world as *excitotoxins* because of their ability to stimulate nerve cells in the brain to rapidly fire and overwork.[7] While some excitotoxins naturally occur in the body, people who consume processed foods are exposed to much greater amounts. The most widely used food addditives that have excitotoxic activity are:

monosodium glutamate,

Rarely does the conventional food industry have your health first and foremost in mind, and they will often use manipulative language on labels to sway your shopping habits.

Certain food additives that enhance flavor are actually known in the science world as excitotoxins because of their ability to stimulate nerve cells in the brain to rapidly fire and overwork. While some excitotoxins naturally occur in the body, people who consume processed foods are exposed to much greater amounts.

Another clue for determining if a food is comprised of whole grains is to read the fiber content. In general, a refined carbohydrate product will have a low fiber content—zero to two grams per serving—for example, while a whole grain product will generally have three grams or more of fiber per serving. Whole grain products will also have higher amounts of protein.

aspartame,

Nutrasweet®,

Equal®, and

hydrolyzed vegetable protein.

These chemical additives are not real food, and they add no nutritional benefit to the diet.

Step 2: Nutrition Facts

After reading the ingredient list and identifying what is in the food product, look more closely at the Nutrition Facts to learn more about the fat, carbohydrate, protein, and vitamin and mineral content of the food. Keep the following in mind when reading the Nutrition Facts:

Servings Per Container

Although a food item may appear to be one serving by itself, such as one small bag of chips, one soda or juice, a can of soup, or one pastry, it will often contain more than one serving. If a package has two servings in it and the whole item is being consumed, one would multiply the number of grams of fat, fiber, and protein as well as the calories by the total number of servings in the package—in this case, times two, to understand the total number of nutrients and calories consumed.

Fat

Recommended dietary fat intake can vary greatly based on the individual, ranging from 75 to 100 grams a day for a 2,000 calorie per day diet. It is helpful to become familiar with which food sources are rich in fat, whether saturated or unsaturated. To give a reference point, a tablespoon of butter, which is a common serving size, has 11 grams of fat, of which 7 grams are saturated. Compare this to a tablespoon of extra virgin olive oil, which has 14 grams of fat, 11 grams of which are monounsaturated. When reading the label, the amount of fat per serving is not as important as the source and quality of fat in the food, which is information you learn from the ingredient list.

Carbohydrates and Fiber

Similar to fat, recommended dietary intake of carbohydrates can vary greatly among individuals based on need, ranging from a low carb intake of 100 grams daily upwards to 300 grams daily. It is helpful to become familiar with carbohydrate-rich food. Recall that sugar and fiber are both sources of carbohydrates. We will dive deeper into understanding the sugar section on the food label in the upcoming **Exploring Sweeteners** chapter. The fiber content listed per serving on the label can actually help you to determine if a food product consists of whole grains. In general, a refined carbohydrate product will have a low fiber content—0 to 2 grams per serving—for example, while a whole grain product will generally have 3 grams or more of fiber per serving. Whole grain products will also have higher amounts of protein. Can you tell from looking at Label 4 and Label 5 which product is whole grain and which is refined?

Label 4 lists *wheat flour* and not whole wheat flour. In addition, it uses *degerminated yellow corn meal*, meaning it has taken out the germ of the grain, thus making it a refined grain product. While Label 5 lists seven whole grains and shows 8 grams of fiber per serving, it also includes multiple types of sweeteners: brown rice syrup, dried cane syrup, and honey, in addition to highly processed canola oil and soy flakes. This adds up to 13 grams of sweetener in 1 cup. Although it is a whole grain product, it is packing a lot of added sugar!

Protein

Visit the protein section to determine if the food provides a good source of protein in your meal planning. Considering that most adults generally need anywhere from 60 to 100 grams of protein a day, a good rule of thumb is to aim for 20 to 30 grams of protein per meal. You can determine if a serving will provide a decent addition to your protein intake or if you need to supplement with another protein-rich food.

Vitamins and Minerals

Packaged foods producers will add vitamins and minerals to their foods (see Label 6) in order to market their products as having higher

Label 4

Nutrition Facts

Serving Size   1/4 Cup (38g/1.3 oz.)
Servings Per Container   About 6

Amount Per Serving	
Calories 170	Calories from Fat 50

	% Daily Value*
Total Fat 4.5g	7%
Saturated Fat 2g	9%
Trans Fat 0g	0%
Polyunsaturated Fat 1g	0%
Monounsaturated Fat 1g	0%
Cholesterol <5mg	1%
Sodium 340mg	14%
Total Carbohydrate 27g	9%
Dietary Fiber <1g	2%
Sugars 7g	
Protein 2g	

Vitamin A 0%	•	Vitamin C 0%
Calcium 8%	•	Iron 6%

INGREDIENTS: WHEAT FLOUR, DEGERMINATED YELLOW CORN MEAL, SUGAR, ANIMAL SHORTENING (CONTAINS ONE OR MORE OF THE FOLLOWING: LARD, HYDROGENATED LARD, PARTIALLY HYDROGENATED LARD), CONTAINS LESS THAN 2% OF EACH OF THE FOLLOWING: BAKING SODA, SODIUM ACID PYROPHOSPHATE, SALT, MONOCALCIUM PHOSPHATE,

Label 5

Nutrition Facts

Serving Size   1 Cup (53g/1.9 oz.)
Servings Per Container   About 7

Amount Per Serving

Calories 200 Calories from Fat 30	
	% Daily Value*
Total Fat 3g	5%
Saturated Fat 0g	0%
Trans Fat 0g	0%
Polyunsaturated Fat 1g	0%
Monounsaturated Fat 1g	0%
Cholesterol 0mg	0%
Sodium 100mg	4%
Potassium 320mg	9%
Total Carbohydrate 38g	13%
Dietary Fiber 8g	33%
Soluble Fiber 8g	
Insoluble Fiber 2g	
Sugars 13g	
Protein 9g	13%
Vitamin A 0% • Vitamin C 0%	
Calcium 2% • Iron 6%	
Phosphorus 10% • Magnesium 10%	

INGREDIENTS: SEVEN WHOLE GRAINS & SESAME BLEND (WHOLE HARD RED WHEAT, BROWN RICE, BARLEY, TRITICALE, OATS, RYE, BUCKWHEAT, SESAME SEEDS), SOY FLAKES, BROWN RICE SYRUP, DRIED CANE SYRUP, CHICORY ROOT FIBER, WHOLE GRAIN OATS, EXPELLER PRESSED CANOLA OIL, HONEY, SALT, CINNAMON, MIXED TOCOPHEROLS FOR FRESHNESS.

Label 6

Nutrition Facts
Serving Size   1 Cup (29g)

Amount Per Serving	Cereal	with ½ cup skim milk
Calories	110	150
Calories from Fat	10	10
	% Daily Value**	
Total Fat 1g*	2%	2%
Saturated Fat 0.5g	3%	3%
Trans Fat 0g		
Polyunsaturated Fat 0g		
Monounsaturated Fat 0g		
Cholesterol 0mg	0%	0%
Sodium 135mg	6%	8%
Potassium 35mg	1%	7%
Total Carbohydrate 26g	9%	11%
Dietary Fiber 3g	10%	10%
Sugars 12g		
Protein 1g		
Vitamin A	10%	15%
Vitamin C	25%	25%
Calcium	0%	15%
Iron	25%	25%
Vitamin D	10%	25%
Thiamin	25%	30%
Riboflavin	25%	35%
Niacin	25%	25%
Vitamin B$_6$	25%	25%
Folic Acid	25%	25%
Vitamin B$_{12}$	25%	35%
Zinc	10%	15%

* Amount in cereal. One half cup of skim milk contributes an additional 40 calories, 65mg sodium, 6g total carbohydrate (6g sugars), and 4g protein.
** Percent Daily Values are based on a 2,000 calorie diet. Your daily values may be higher or lower depending on your calorie needs:

	Calories	2,000	2,500
Total Fat	Less than	65g	80g
Sat. Fat	Less than	20g	25g
Cholesterol	Less than	300mg	300mg
Sodium	Less than	2,400mg	2,400mg
Potassium		3,500mg	3,500mg
Total Carbohydrate		300g	375g
Dietary Fiber		25g	30g

Ingredients: Sugar, corn flour blend (whole grain yellow corn flour, degerminated yellow corn flour), wheat flour, whole grain oat flour, oat fiber, soluble corn fiber, contains 2% or less of partially hydrogenated vegetable oil (coconut, soybean and/or cottonseed), salt, red 40, natural flavor, blue 2, turmeric color, yellow 6, annatto color, blue 1, BHT for freshness.

Vitamins and Minerals: Vitamin C (sodium ascorbate and ascorbic acid), niacinamide, reduced iron, zinc oxide, vitamin B$_6$ (pyridoxine hydrochloride), vitamin B$_2$ (riboflavin), vitamin B$_1$ (thiamin hydrochloride), vitamin A palmitate, folic acid, vitamin D, vitamin B$_{12}$.

CONTAINS WHEAT INGREDIENTS. CORN USED IN THIS PRODUCT MAY CONTAIN TRACES OF SOYBEANS.

nutritional value. Don't be fooled. Some of these products may still have high amounts of sugar, trans fats, and refined carbohydrates. Rest assured that if your diet includes frequent and diverse fresh fruits and vegetables, whole grains, and legumes, there will be little to no benefit to eating highly processed foods with added vitamins and minerals.

Sodium

Salt is composed of two minerals called sodium and chloride. Many packaged and processed foods contain high amounts of sodium to tantalize our taste buds, as well as for food preservation. For some people, excess sodium in the diet can contribute to high blood pressure, cardiovascular, and kidney disease. On the other hand, strictly limiting sodium intake also has it own health risks.[8] What is the recommended daily intake of sodium? Most major medical organizations recommend approximately 5.8 grams of salt per day, which equals about **2,300 mg of sodium/day** or **one teaspoon of table salt**.[9,10] It is not difficult to go over this limit by consuming many boxed and canned goods. Decreasing boxed and packaged food use is the easiest way to avoid excess sodium, as well as chemical additives and BPA (Bisphenol A), which will be discussed soon. However, if that is not possible, consider rinsing and straining canned vegetables and beans to decrease the sodium content.

Label Reading In Action

When you think of peanut butter, imagine what ingredients you would expect to actually be in peanut butter. Most people would say *ground peanuts*. Yet, Popular Peanut Butter One has added sugar and a blend of three types of highly processed and poor quality hydrogenated oils. The Nutrition Facts information is actually quite comparable between the two different types of peanut butters, but the level of processing between the brands is quite different. Popular Peanut Butter Two contains only two, simple ingredients. You wouldn't be able to see that information just by looking at the numbers in the Nutrition Facts section.

The following labels compare two popular peanut butters:

Popular Peanut Butter One

Nutrition Facts

Serving Size   2 Tbsp (32g)
Servings Per Container About 14

Amount Per Serving

Calories 190   Calories from Fat 140

	% Daily Value*
Total Fat 16g	25%
Saturated Fat 3g	15%
Trans Fat 0g	0%
Polyunsaturated Fat 1g	0%
Monounsaturated Fat 1g	0%
Cholesterol 0mg	0%
Sodium 125mg	5%
Total Carbohydrate 7g	2%
Dietary Fiber 2g	8%
Sugars 3g	
Protein 7g	7%

Vitamin A 0%	•	Vitamin C 0%
Calcium 2%	•	Iron 4%
Vitamin E 10%	•	Niacin 20%

INGREDIENTS: ROASTED PEANUTS, SUGAR, HYDROGENATED VEGETABLE OILS (COTTONSEED, SOYBEAN, RAPESEED) TO PREVENT SEPARATION: SALT.

Popular Peanut Butter Two

Nutrition Facts

Serving Size   2 Tbsp (32g)
Servings Per Container About 14

Amount Per Serving

Calories 180   Calories from Fat 140

	% Daily Value*
Total Fat 15g	23%
Saturated Fat 2g	11%
Trans Fat 0g	0%
Polyunsaturated Fat 1g	0%
Monounsaturated Fat 1g	0%
Cholesterol 0mg	0%
Sodium 60mg	3%
Total Carbohydrate 6g	3%
Dietary Fiber 2g	8%
Sugars 1g	
Protein 8g	8%

Vitamin A 0%	•	Vitamin C 0%
Calcium 0%	•	Iron 0%
Vitamin E 10%	•	Niacin 20%

INGREDIENTS: ORGANIC DRY ROASTED PEANUTS, SEA SALT

While we do not promote calorie-counting as a healthy way to relate to whole foods, it is helpful to get a baseline education about which foods and drinks tend to be highly caloric. These foods tend to be high in fat or added sweeteners. Knowing that most adults typically consume from 1500 to 2500 calories a day, you can reference how this food or drink fits into a typical daily caloric intake.

To practice some of the steps that we have outlined, start reading labels that you already have at home. Find three products with food labels to review the following and practice the steps we've outlined. Some ideas of labels to look at are: a box of cereal, peanut butter, a loaf of bread, or a can of soup.

Determine the following from the Ingredients list:

Would you consider this to be a whole food product or a highly processed food?

What are the sources of added sweeteners and how much has been added?

Are there any trans fats? How do you know?

Is this food a good source of fiber?

Does it contain any chemical additives?

Next, identify the following on the food label section, Nutrition Facts:

Serving size. Does this appear to be a reasonable serving size, or are you likely to eat or drink more than one serving?

Servings per container. Be sure to multiply all Nutrition Facts quantities by the number of serving sizes if you are going to consume the entire container.

Calories. While we do not promote calorie counting as a healthy way to relate to whole foods, it is helpful to get a baseline education about which foods and drinks tend to be highly caloric. These foods tend to be high in fat or added sweeteners. Knowing that most adults typically consume from 1500 to 2500 calories a day, you can reference how this food or drink fits into a typical daily caloric intake.

Calories from Fat. Compare to total calories to determine if this is a fat-rich food.

Percent Daily Value (%DV). This value helps you determine if a food or drink is high or low in a particular nutrient. Food or drink providing more than 20% of (%DV) can be considered a rich source and less than 5% a low source.

Total Fat. A total daily intake of fat can vary greatly between individuals, ranging from 75 to 100 grams, for example. Determine if a serving size of this food contributes a rich source of dietary fat.

Saturated Fat. If the food contains grams of saturated fat, read the ingredient list to find out if it comes from a plant or animal source.

Unsaturated Fat. Often the label will differentiate the grams of polyunsaturated versus monounsaturated fats.

Trans Fat. Remember that a food may contain trans fats even if it lists 0 grams on the Nutrition Facts label. Read the ingredient list of the label to identify any *partially hydrogenated* oils.

Cholesterol. Cholesterol-rich foods come from animals. A serving size containing more than 100 mg of cholesterol can be considered a cholesterol-rich food.

Sodium. Pay attention to how many servings you plan on consuming to determine your total sodium intake.

Total Carbohydrates. Individuals vary greatly with their daily carb intake, ranging from a low-carb intake of 100 grams daily upwards to 300 grams daily. Determine if eating a serving size or two will contribute significantly to your daily intake.

Dietary Fiber. Fiber rich foods tend to have 3 grams or more per serving.

Sugar. In 2014, the FDA proposed changes to the Nutrition Facts label that would require listing the amount of added versus naturally occurring sugar in a food. Until these changes take effect, it is up to the consumer to identify and calculate the amounts of naturally occurring sugars and added sugars. We will learn this skill in Chapter Nine, **Exploring Sweeteners**.

Protein. We mentioned earlier the wide variation in individual protein requirements, from 50 to 175 grams daily. A general guideline for most adults is to consume 20 to 30 grams of protein per meal. Determine if a serving size of this food will be a good contribution.

Vitamins and Minerals. Use the %DV to determine if this food or drink is a rich source of a particular vitamin or mineral. Check the ingredient list to determine if the food or drink has been enriched with added vitamins or minerals or if they are naturally occurring.

In 2014, the FDA proposed changes to the Nutrition Facts label that would require listing the amount of added, versus naturally occurring, sugar in a food. Until these changes take effect, it is up to the consumer to identify and calculate the amounts of naturally occurring sugars and added sugars.

Common Label Claims and Certifications

Now that you know how to read the most important part of a food label—the **Ingredients** list, and you know how to navigate the **Nutrition Facts**, let us focus on some of the claims and labeling that might be found on the front of a label, can, jar, or box.

Labels Regulated by the Federal Government

Organic

Foods labeled *organic* have been certified by a third party agency. The term generally signifies that the plants or animals have been grown or raised without the use of pesticides and with seeds that are not genetically modified. Technically, *organic* should mean it is a non-GMO food; yet it is difficult to test the seeds regularly and instances of contamination are becoming more common.

Organic meat or poultry is livestock that are fed organic feed without any animal by-products. They are not given any growth hormones or antibiotics. In addition, the meats must not be irradiated. The animals must also be given access to the outdoors, but the *organic* label does not distinguish the amount of time the animals spend outside or the amount of space they can access.

Consider the following as you navigate whether or not to purchase organic foods.

Benefits of purchasing organic foods:

- decreased exposure to toxic chemicals,
- decreased risk of allergic reactions to chemicals and pesticides on food,
- increased nutrient quality of food, specifically antioxidants,[11]
- better for the environment, and
- decreased toxic exposure to farm workers.

Additional purchasing factors to consider:

- possible increased cost of organic foods,
- availability, and

Foods labeled organic have been certified by a third party agency. The term generally signifies that the plants or animals have been grown or raised without the use of pesticides and with seeds that are not genetically modified.

- difficulty of local farmers to be certified *organic* due to cost of the certification. (Buying local, non-organic food may still provide you with an option for pesticide-free produce. Talk to your local farmers about their food production practices.)

The Environmental Working Group is an independent organization that rates fresh produce annually according to their residual pesticide content. If you are just starting to purchase organic produce, we recommend using the *Dirty Dozen* and *Clean Fifteen* list for shopping to help you navigate what foods to purchase organic.

The list is updated every year, but to give you an example of what you might find, the *2015 Dirty Dozen* (high amount of pesticide residue on fresh produce) includes: apples, peaches, nectarines, strawberries, grapes, celery, spinach, sweet bell peppers, cucumber, cherry tomatoes, snap peas, potatoes, hot peppers, kale, and collard greens.

The *2015 Clean Fifteen* (lowest amount of pesticide residue on fresh produce) includes: avocados, sweet corn, pineapples, cabbage, sweet peas, onions, asparagus, mangos, papayas, kiwi, eggplant, grapefruit, cantaloupe, cauliflower, and sweet potatoes.

Free-Range

The term, free-range, is regulated by the USDA for poultry—chicken, turkey, and duck, for example. Free-range means that the animals have had access to the outdoors. However, this definition can be loosely interpreted and farms are often not regularly inspected. Some farms may allow the chickens to roam freely in a large pasture for most of the day, returning to the indoors only at night. Because the term does not address the population density or the quality of the outdoor experience, it could mean they have a small area of dirt or gravel, having to stand with minimal movement due to crowding.

Labels Not Regulated by the Federal Government

Grass-Fed

As of January 2016, the term "grass-fed" is no longer regulated by the USDA for beef. Grass-fed refers to cattle that have only been eating grass or hay and are not being fed grain or animal by-products.

The Environmental Working Group is an independent organization that rates fresh produce annually according to their residual pesticide content. If you are just starting to purchase organic produce, we recommend using the Dirty Dozen *and* Clean Fifteen *list for shopping to help you navigate what foods to purchase organic.*

*The word, natural, on a food product may be the most confusing and misleading food label claim. Generally speaking, a food labeled as natural, with the exception of meat and poultry, may not carry much weight. Broadly, it means that the food was minimally processed and free of synthetic additives, but this label is not subject to government controls. Some cereals, condiments, breads, soups, or peanut butters are labeled as **All Natural**. Look deeper into the **Ingredients** list to be sure it is not just a marketing strategy.*

Grass-fed cattle have access to large areas of pasture to roam and graze on their natural grass diet. Compared to conventional beef, meat from cattle raised on a grass-based diet is leaner and more nutritious, with increased total conjugated linoleic acid (CLA), a precursor to a form of anti-inflammatory omega-6 fatty acids, and omega-3 fatty acids. In addition, it also contains higher amounts of beta-carotene and vitamin E, as well as cancer-fighting antioxidants such as glutathione and superoxide dismutase.[12] However, even with this label, there can be confusion. Cattle may be grass-fed for a portion of their lives and then be fed processed corn and soy in order for them to gain weight quickly before being processed into meat. If you want to determine if the cattle were grass-fed for their entire lives, you can look for labels such as *100% grass-fed* and *grass-finished*.

Cage-free

There are no legal definitions for *cage-free*. You may find this label on chicken, turkey, or more commonly, eggs. It means the chickens were not raised in cages. It does not necessarily mean that they had access to the outdoors or even access to large areas indoors.

Pasture-raised

Another unregulated term, *pasture-raised,* generally signifies that the animal had access to outdoor pastures (not gravel or dirt) in order to freely roam and graze for food. You might find this label on eggs, butter, poultry, and beef.

Natural

The word, *natural,* on a food product may be the most confusing and misleading food label claim. Generally speaking, a food labeled as *natural*, with the exception of meat and poultry, may not carry much weight. Broadly, it means that the food was minimally processed and free of synthetic additives, but this label is not subject to government controls. Some cereals, condiments, breads, soups, or peanut butters are labeled as *All Natural*. Look deeper into the **Ingredients** list to be sure it is not just a marketing strategy.

However, meat and poultry that are labeled *natural are* regulated by the federal government. In these cases, it means that the product should be free of artificial colors, flavors, sweeteners, and preservatives. Natural meat and poultry must be minimally processed and not altered from the original raw product. Remember, *natural meat* on a label represents little to do with what the animal was fed or what environment the animal was raised in; it is **only** referring to the processing of the animal.

Genetically Modified Organisms (GMOs)

Genetically engineered or modified organisms (GMOs) were introduced into the environment about thirty years ago, ultimately allowing technology to alter and add genetic material into our food supply. These foods are created in a laboratory and have not evolved naturally. Up to 70% of packaged foods in the USA may contain ingredients from the three most commonly genetically modified foods: corn, soy, and canola.[13] We strongly question the role of GMO food in a low-processed, whole foods diet. As of 2015, there is currently no requirement in the United States to label genetically modified or engineered foods. This is in stark contrast to at least sixty-four countries around the world, including the European Union, Russia, China, Japan, and Australia, that have banned, restricted, or required labeling of GMOs.

Our concern with GMO foods is the lack of long-term studies examining their effects on human and environmental health. For instance, a gene from a Brazil nut, when transferred into a soybean, has been shown to elicit an allergic reaction in people with a nut allergy.[14] Additionally, there is cause for concern regarding the unpredictable contamination of organic crops with GMOs as well as the impact of GMO on the health of insect pollinators.[15] The *Non-GMO Project* is the only independent organization in the United States and Canada that verifies that a product is at least 99.1% GMO -free, with the aim of 100%. They routinely test ingredients at high risk of GMO contamination and ensure that the company is following best practices for continued avoidance of GMO contamination.

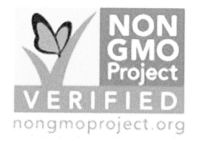

The Non-GMO Project *is the only independent organization in the United States and Canada that verifies that a product is at least 99.1% GMO-free, with the aim of 100%.*

Look for a label and seal that says *Non-GMO Project Verified*. If you see the general label, *GMO-Free*, know that it may not have been verified by a third party.

Whole Grains Stamp

The Whole Grains Council verifies if a food product is a good source of whole grains or if it is a 100% whole grain product. A food product with the basic stamp contains at least half a serving (8 grams) of whole grains, but it may also still contain refined grains. The 100% whole grain stamp identifies products that are made completely with whole grains, including the bran, endosperm, and germ.

Not all food companies are using the whole grain stamp; but as we previously outlined above, you can determine if a product is a whole grain product by reading the ingredient list.

BPA-Free (Bisphenol-A)

Certain canned foods are noting on their label that they are *BPA-free*. BPA is a chemical that is commonly used in the inner lining of canned goods such as soups, tomatoes, beans, vegetables, and fruits. It has also commonly been used in many plastic goods such as bottled water, juice, soda, baby bottles, plastic toys, and the lining of sales receipts. The concern is that BPA leaches out of these products and can ultimately be absorbed into the body. BPA is considered an *endocrine disruptor* due to its similar chemical structure to one of the natural estrogens produced in the human body. Thus, it can bind and activate the same receptors as natural estrogens and can affect hormone biochemistry. Exposure to BPA may contribute to thyroid, nervous, and reproductive system dysfunction, as well as affect hormonally-influenced cancers, such as breast and prostate.[16,17]

Canada was the first country to declare BPA a toxic substance. In 2012, the Food and Drug Administration banned BPA use in baby bottles and sippy cups but has not gone so far as to say that the chemical is toxic or harmful. Despite lack of government action, companies are moving away from using BPA in their products due to consumer demand. Unfortunately, some of the chemicals that manufacturers

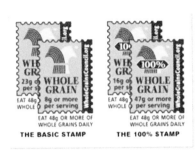

THE BASIC STAMP   THE 100% STAMP

The Whole Grains Council verifies if a food product is a good source of whole grains or if it is a 100% whole grain product. A food product with the basic stamp contains at least half a serving (8 grams) of whole grains, but it may also still contain refined grains. The 100% whole grain stamp identifies products that are made completely with whole grains, including the bran, endosperm, and germ.

are using instead of BPA may turn out to be just as harmful. The bottom line is to generally avoid food and drink packaged in plastic and to shop around for alternative packaging. Tomato sauce, crushed tomatoes, salad dressings, condiments such as mustard, sauces, oils, and vinegar are sold in glass jars. You can wash and reuse the glass containers to store your bulk items. Otherwise, look for the BPA-free label.

Congratulations! You are ready to hit the aisles with your new label reading skills! Remember: reading the ingredient list is *the* most important thing to do when becoming a conscientious shopper. We also recommend expanding your food shopping experiences by visiting local health food stores and farmers' markets. Don't be afraid to ask where the food came from and how it was grown or raised. Many local farms welcome visitors, and you can see firsthand how produce is grown and animals are raised. Because of the lack of clarity in food label claims, including cage-free and free-range, having a direct conversation with the person who raised the animals can clear up much confusion.

Keep in mind that some small farmers cannot afford certifications like *organic* for their food labels. Smaller farming operations are often growing food organically and in a more natural environment than some of the large-scale farms that do the bare minimum to achieve and afford certification. Talk to your local farmers directly to learn about their growing practices.

We hope you become inspired to learn more about what is in your food and where it comes from. The next time you are out food shopping, make the best decision you can with your new knowledge and skills regarding whole foods. Then, return home and create and enjoy simple, delicious meals. You are well on your way to reclaiming your health with whole foods.

BPA is considered an **endocrine disruptor** *due to its similar chemical structure to one of the natural estrogens produced in the human body. Thus, it can bind and activate the same receptors as natural estrogens and can affect hormone biochemistry. Exposure to BPA may contribute to thyroid, nervous, and reproductive system dysfunction, as well as affect hormonally influenced cancers, such as breast and prostate.*

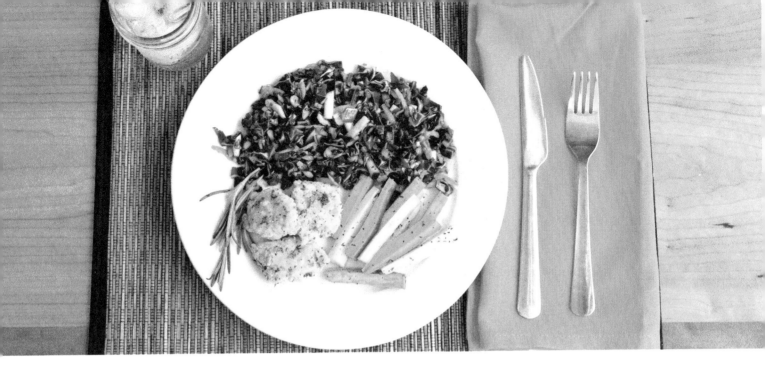

CHAPTER SIX

The FAME Plate

Since I was 13, I have tried dozens of diets (Atkins®, Weight Watchers®, and Nutri-System® to name a few). I find it very comforting to know that I really can't go wrong with whole foods and a well balanced plate with greens, whole grains, protein, and fats. I will never go to the grocery store again without examining a label, buying a leafy green, and thinking of FAME!

—Allison, FAME series, Charlee's Kitchen

THE AMOUNT OF FOOD COMMONLY SERVED AT A RESTAURANT HAS DRAMATICALLY INCREASED OVER THE LAST 10 TO 20 YEARS. Think about the enormous pasta portions served in many Italian restaurants. Consider the sheer volume of a 32-ounce Big Gulp® soda or a 20-ounce Venti® latte. This notion of *bigger is better* has paralleled our worsening health. Bottomless sodas, super-size French fries, and *free* baskets of bread have become the norm when eating out. At grocery stores, nutrient-poor, highly processed foods such as chips, crackers, and frozen food are sold in greater quantities at lower prices due to bulk packaging and cheap ingredients. While this may be convenient and economical to the consumer, it often promotes increased consumption of low-quality foods at a cost to health.

Large portion sizes have been connected with metabolic syndrome, insulin resistance, and obesity.[1] Research shows that limiting (or using appropriate) portion sizes will decrease food intake.[2] By creating the healthy habit of understanding and using appropriate portion sizes, we are less likely to consume excess food.

Serving Size Versus Portion Size

The **serving sizes** that are on the Nutrition Facts label are standardized measurements of food that are set by the USDA Center for Nutrition Policy and Promotion. A **portion size** is the amount of food that is *actually* consumed in one sitting.

In the past thirty years, **the portions consumed in America have nearly doubled in size.** People are often unaware that packaged food, bottled drinks, and restaurant meals often contain more than one serving.

For example, the Dietary Guidelines suggest that a standard bagel serving size is two ounces, yet the average bagel sold is six ounces. Most people will eat a whole bagel as a portion, thus eating *three* servings. This doesn't mean you cannot enjoy a modern-size bagel. Just be aware that there are multiple servings in the portion size. The point is, Americans are eating more than they ever have and restaurants and grocery stores are pushing the idea that bigger is better.

Nutritional Guidelines And Healthy Plates

The federal government (USDA) promotes MyPlate, a nutritional guideline using a plate as a visual aid to create healthy meals. There are many examples of *healthy plates* created by various nutrition organizations and educational institutions. Our concern is that many other guidelines still promote the consumption of refined grains and highly processed oils like soybean, corn, canola, and even margarine, which often contain trans fats.

The plate we present to you focuses on whole foods and allows for variation from person to person. A person may need less carbohydrates or more protein, for example, depending on what is best for his

20 years ago		Today
3 in	Bagel	6 in
8 oz	Soda	20 oz
8 oz	Coffee	16 oz
5 cups	Popcorn	20 cups
500 Calories	Pizza	850 Calories

or her body's needs. A person's ethical choices in regard to animal products will also affect what is necessary for a healthy plate.

We will start with *what* food to include on your plate and then look at *how* much.

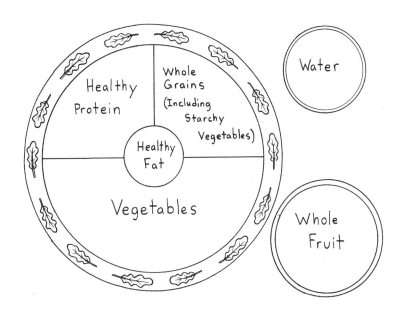

The FAME Plate

The following steps will help you learn how a dinner, lunch, or breakfast plate would look with food in healthy portions:

1. Use a normal-sized plate: approximately 10.5 to 11 inches in diameter. Measure the plate. Plates are sometimes up to 14 inches in diameter, which may also make it more difficult to eat appropriate portions.

2. Fill half (½) the plate with non-starchy vegetables.
    Examples: all dark green leafy vegetables (spinach, chard, kale, collards), lettuce, broccoli, bok choy, cauliflower, onion, garlic, leeks, Brussels sprouts, carrots, celery, asparagus, bell peppers, cucumber, tomato (fruit), mushroom.

3. Fill one-fourth (¼) of the plate with whole grains and/or starchy vegetables.
    Examples: all whole grains including brown rice, corn, quinoa, oats, and whole grain pasta or whole grain bread. Starchy vegetables such as yams, sweet potato, beets, or squash.

4. Fill one-fourth (¼) of the plate with a low-processed source of protein.

   Examples: meat, poultry, wild game, fish, eggs, dairy, beans, nuts and nut butters, seeds.

5. The middle circle targets the inclusion of healthy fats and oils.

   Examples: avocado, coconut or coconut oil, olives or olive oil, butter and other full-fat dairy, nuts and nut butters, egg yolk, lard and tallow.

6. Whole Fruit: includes berries, pears, apples, citrus, melons, grapes.

7. Beverage: drink water!

Tips For Creating The FAME Plate

- Fruit does not *need* to be eaten at every meal, but is definitely part of a healthy diet and can be used in a meal or as a snack. The general trend is that Americans disproportionately choose fruits over vegetables. To bring back balance, note how much more space vegetables have on the FAME Plate. Fill half (½) your plate with vegetables and you'll be on the right track!

- Notice that most foods contain a combination of macronutrients (fats, carbs, and protein) and may fit into more than one category. Quinoa is a complete protein, but it is also a good source of complex carbohydrates. Beans are the same way: high in fiber and protein. Nuts are high in protein and healthy fats. While the FAME Plate has separate sections, whole foods fall into more than one nutrient category. Place a food into the category it fits best for each meal.

- The FAME Plate is only a guideline, and it doesn't need to be a perfect science. If one gets overly focused on the details, the big picture of moving toward a whole foods diet may be

*The **FAME Plate** is only a guideline, and it doesn't need to be a perfect science. If one gets overly focused on the details, the big picture of moving toward a whole foods diet may be lost. Remember, each person has an individual relationship with food based on many factors including family and cultural traditions, food allergies or sensitivities, and health goals. Therefore, food groups and portions may be individualized.*

lost. Remember, each person has an individual relationship with food based on many factors including family and cultural traditions, food allergies or sensitivities, and health goals. Therefore, food groups and portions may be individualized.

What About Dairy?

Unlike some plate models, dairy does not get its own section on the FAME Plate. It is part of a healthy diet for some people as a source of protein *and* fat and can be used in those sections of the plate. It does not need to be included in every meal, as it is often suggested. People often include dairy as a source of calcium, though research shows this is not the most optimal way to consume this important mineral in the diet.

The dairy industry is hugely successful at marketing its product. Who hasn't seen the infamous milk moustache? People are led to believe that the best, and sometimes only, food that contains calcium is dairy products. There is prolific and constant campaigning from the *Dairy Council* for people to drink three glasses of milk a day to support healthy bones.

It is important to note that this highly marketed milk comes from dairy cows within the industrialized food system. The cows are generally not pasture-raised, thus decreasing the nutritional status of the milk, including decreased beta-carotene, vitamin E, omega-3 fatty acids, and CLA (conjugated linoleic acid).[3,4,5] In addition, the milk is pasteurized, killing the naturally occurring enzymes and probiotics that can help humans digest cow's milk. Dairy can be a detrimental food choice for those with lactose intolerance, a common deficiency in the enzyme lactase, which breaks down milk sugar, as well as those with a dairy allergy or sensitivity.

While it is true that our body needs dietary calcium to build bones, it is often overemphasized. The research looking at dairy intake and fracture risk varies widely and may make you rethink the classic advice to consume large amounts of dairy. *The Harvard Nurses' Study,* which followed more than 75,000 women for twelve years, found that

Unlike some plate models, dairy does not get its own section on the FAME Plate. It is part of a healthy diet for some people as a source of protein and fat and can be used in those sections of the plate. It does not need to be included in every meal, as it is often suggested. People often include dairy as a source of calcium, though research shows this is not the most optimal way to consume this important mineral in the diet.

those who drank three of more glasses of milk a day had no reduction in the risk of hip or arm fractures compared to those who drank little or no milk. These findings emerged after the study took into account the women's weight, tobacco use, alcohol use, and menopausal status. In actuality, increased intake of calcium from dairy products was associated with a higher fracture risk.[6]

Bone health and preventing osteoporosis are more complicated than just looking at calcium. You must assess certain risk factors such as one's family history of osteoporosis, gender, hormone status, a personal history of low body weight, and ancestry. Other factors for prevention of osteoporosis that are just as or more important are regular weight-bearing exercise, sun exposure (or vitamin D intake), and eating a balance of foods rich in vitamin K, calcium, and other minerals. In addition to increased fracture risk, there is also concern and research showing that high intake of dairy products is associated with increased risk and occurrence of ovarian and prostate cancer.[7,8,9,10]

When looking at other sources of calcium besides dairy, you find that not all calcium is created equal. For instance, only 30% of the calcium from dairy is readily absorbed by the digestive tract, while 40 to 64% of the calcium in vegetables like broccoli, Brussels sprouts, mustard greens, turnip greens, and kale is absorbed.[11,12] (Take note that while spinach contains considerable calcium, it is not easily absorbable because of high levels of oxalic acid.) Dairy products contain high amounts of phosphorous, which inhibits the absorption of calcium. This means that although there may be less calcium in plants than in dairy, our body will use it more readily. This is likely due to the synergy and balance among the other vitamins and minerals in the leafy greens. This includes vitamin K, beta-carotene, magnesium, iron, and more, all of which are all needed for bone health.

Here's some good news: that same *Harvard Nurses Study* showed that women eating one serving of lettuce or other green, leafy vegetable a day cut their risk of hip fracture in half when compared with eating one serving a week. Once again we are reminded to eat a variety of vegetables every day. The best sources of plant-based calcium are greens and beans, so enjoy!

All said, dairy foods can be part of a healthy, whole foods diet for those who tolerate dairy. As with anything you are eating, it depends on how much, where it came from, the degree of processing, and in this case, how the animals were raised. The best option would be to choose locally-raised dairy products from organic, pasture-raised cows, sheep, or goats, and to eat dairy in moderation.

Here is a useful guide of calcium levels in common foods. Notice there is more calcium in one cup of cooked collard greens (358 mg) or in 3 ounces of sardines (325 mg) than in one-half cup of whole milk (300 mg).

Table 6.1 Food Sources of Calcium

Food Item	Calcium (mg)
Almonds (¼ cup)	95
Barley (1 cup)	57
Black turtle beans (1 cup, cooked)	103
Bok choy (½ cup, cooked)	79
Broccoli (1 cup, cooked)	94
Brussels sprouts (8 sprouts)	56
Butternut squash (1 cup, cooked)	84
Chick peas (1 cup, cooked)	80
Collard greens (1 cup, cooked)	358
Figs (10 medium, dried)	269
Great northern beans (1 cup, cooked)	121
Green beans (1 cup, cooked)	58
Kale (1 cup, cooked)	94
Lentils (1 cup, cooked)	37
Lima beans (1 cup, cooked)	32
Mustard greens (1 cup, cooked)	150
Navel orange (1 medium)	56
Navy beans (1 cup, cooked)	128
Peas (1 cup, cooked)	44

Table 6.1 Food Sources of Calcium (cont'd)

Food Item	Calcium (mg)
Pink salmon (3 oz, cooked, with bone)	181
Pinto beans (1 cup, cooked)	82
Rhubarb (½ cup, cooked)	174
Sardines (3 oz, Atlantic, in oil, drained)	325
Sesame seeds (1 tablespoon)	90
Spinach (½ cup, cooked)	115
Sweet potato (1 cup, cooked)	70
Tempeh (1 cup)	184
White beans (1 cup, cooked)	161
Whole milk (½ cup)	300

Daily Servings

Exactly how much food should be on the plate? If your plate looks like the FAME Plate at each meal, you are probably doing well maximizing your nutritional intake. Again, this is just a visual guide. Most meals won't have each food perfectly in its section and many foods overlap categories. The food on some plates may fit into the distinct categories and locations on the plate: fish (protein, fat), sautéed vegetables, quinoa (whole grain, protein), and coconut oil (healthy fat). For other meals, the plate might mix all

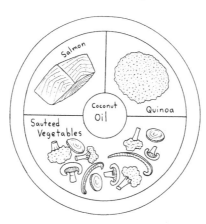

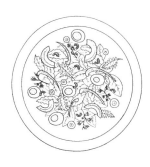

Portion Size Guide

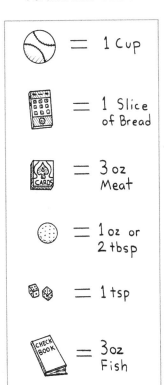

sections together. Consider a big salad with salad greens, carrots, cucumbers (vegetables), with hard-boiled egg, nuts (fat, protein), and avocado and olive oil for dressing (healthy fats).

In addition to *what* foods are on the FAME Plate, it is important to take into account *how much* food should be on the plate at each meal. This amount will ultimately depend on each individual's metabolic needs. But as a starting point for most people, using visual aids and common household items can help in remembering appropriate portions, aside from actually measuring them out. Look at the handy Portion Size Guide.

Here are some examples of portion sizes using the guide as well as suggestions for how to build a healthy plate:

Vegetables

On the FAME Plate, non-starchy vegetables are unlimited. Aim for at least 1½ cups of cooked vegetables or 2 cups of salad greens per meal:

> ½ cup cooked vegetables (5 to 10 grams)= ½ baseball
> 1 cup of salad greens (2 grams) = baseball

Whole Grains And Starchy Vegetables

In the whole grain and starchy vegetable section, include one of the following choices:

> 1 cup starchy vegetables (15 to 27 grams): potato (white or sweet), yam, squash, beets = baseball
> ½ cup of cooked whole grains or pasta (18 to 25 grams)—except oats = ½ baseball
> 1 cup cooked oats (27 grams) = baseball
> 1 slice of whole grain bread (12 grams) = size of smart phone

Note that in the case of a sandwich, you may be consuming 2 to 3 portions of whole grains. The key is to consider your diet in general and create balance as much as possible. Enjoy the sandwich, but consider eating less carb-rich foods at the next meal.

Protein

Protein intake depends on body size and individual metabolic needs. Include one of the following at each meal:

  3 to 4 ounces of meat, poultry, wild game (20 to 25 grams) = deck of cards, palm of hand

  3 to 4 ounces of fish (20 to 25 grams) = checkbook

If choosing vegetarian or plant-based proteins, chose 2 to 3 of the following for each meal:

  ¼ cup of nuts or seeds (5-8 grams) = small handful

  2 tablespoons of nut butters (7 to 8 grams) = ping pong ball

  ½ cup cooked beans and legumes (7 to 8 grams) = ½ baseball

  ½ cup high protein whole grains, such as amaranth or quinoa (7 to 8 grams) = 1/2 baseball

  1 egg (7 to 8 grams)

  1 cup of whole milk or yogurt (8 grams) = baseball

  1 to 1½ ounces of cheese (8 grams) = 2 dice

Fats and Oils

Include 1 to 2 sources of healthy fat per meal:

  1 tablespoon butter or oil (coconut, olive oil) (11 to 16 grams) = 2 dice

  ½ medium avocado (11 to 15 grams)

  ¼ cup of nuts or seeds (14 grams) = small handful

  1 cup olives (15 grams)

  3 tablespoons shedded coconut (10 grams)

  ¼ cup full-fat coconut milk (12 grams)

  1 cup whole milk or yogurt (9 grams)

  1½ ounces of cheese (13 to 15 grams)

Fruits

While it is optional to include fruit at every meal, you can include 1 to 3 of the following in meals or snacks throughout the day:

  1 medium-sized whole fruit = 1 baseball

  ½ cup of fresh cut fruit = ½ baseball

  ¼ cup dried or dehydrated fruit (no sugar added, preservative free) = size of egg

Tips For Creating Appropriate Portions

When Buying Bulk

- Re-package oversized foods into appropriate-sized containers.

When Eating Out

- Split your entrée with a friend or family member.
- Ask to have half the entrée boxed to go and eat it for a meal the next day.
- Skip the "free" bread or chips served before the meal.
- Avoid appetizers. They tend to be high-calorie and nutrient-poor food. Order a salad as an appetizer instead.
- Substitute French fries, chips, or other refined carbohydrate–rich side dishes for vegetables. Most restaurants offer a salad or sautéed vegetables.
- Keep it simple if traveling or eating out regularly for work. Order salad or vegetables with a source of protein.
- Ask if there is a small or kid-size portion for occasional fried foods or desserts.

When Eating At Home

- Serve meals onto plates according to the FAME Plate method and keep the serving dishes away from the table.
- Only eat *seconds* if choosing vegetables.
- Never combine eating snacks *out of the bag* with watching TV. Guess what happens?
- If hunger strikes and lunch or dinner is a couple of hours away, first drink a glass of water and wait 10 minutes. Dehydration can often mimic hunger. If hungry still, eat a small healthy snack (like a small handful of nuts or carrots or celery with hummus, for example) to avoid overeating at mealtime.
- When choosing the right whole foods that are balanced in protein, fats, and carbohydrates, as well as eating in a way that encourages healthy digestion, the body will tell you when full and satisfied. Listen closely.

USDA Guidelines For Caloric Intake Compared To Current Research To Support Healthy Metabolism And Weight Loss

While we are not promoting any specific *diet* to our readers nor do we emphasize calorie counting as a sustainable way to relate to food, we do think it is important to compare what the United States Department of Agriculture presents as a proper breakdown of caloric intake compared to other points of view that medical experts have supported. The USDA's version is presented on most food labels and therefore is most familiar to American eaters.

Table 6.2 USDA Guidelines for Daily Caloric Intake

Nutrients	2,000 Calories Per Day	2,500 Calories Per Day
Total fat (F)	Less than 65 g (30% of daily calories)	80 g (30%)
Total carbohydrates (C)	300 g (60% of daily calories)	375 g (60%)
Dietary fiber	25 g	30 g
Protein (P)	50 grams/day (10% of daily calories)	62.5 g (10%)

Take a moment to consider a popular meal of pasta and meat sauce based upon the USDA model for someone eating three meals a day. It may look like this:

One-third (4 ounces) of a standard whole wheat spaghetti box
   (This amount of pasta is also equivalent to two serving sizes of pasta).
½ cup pasta sauce
2 ounces pork sausage

Total: Carbohydrates (100 grams) + Fat (18 grams) +Protein (23 grams) + 15 grams of fiber

The carbohydrate-rich pasta would be the predominant feature on the plate. The USDA model is carbohydrate heavy, with a recommended intake of 60% of daily calories from carbohydrates. Research is growing to suggest that a low-glycemic diet, or a diet that contains a lower percentage of calories from carbohydrates, can better support metabolism for weight loss goals, weight loss maintenance, and reduced risk of metabolic disorders like diabetes and metabolic syndrome.[13] A healthy plate based on low-glycemic foods would have a lower percentage of daily calories coming from carbohydrates (approximately 40%) and a higher percentage coming from proteins and healthy fats (20% and 40% respectively), which is more in alignment with our FAME Plate model. This model also includes a level of daily fiber intake that most naturopathic doctors consider optimal (35 to 50 grams daily).

Table 6.3 Low-glycemic Guidelines for Daily Caloric Intake

Nutrients	2,000 Calories Per Day	2,500 Calories Per Day
Total fat (F)	85-90 g (40% of daily calories)	110 g (40%)
Total carbohydrates (C)	200 g (40% of daily calories)	250 g (40%)
Dietary fiber	35-50 g	35-50 g
Protein (P)	100-105 g (20% of daily calories)	125 g (20%)

Now, let's reconsider the pasta meal, based on the low-glycemic recommendations.

One-sixth (2 ounces) of a standard whole wheat spaghetti box
½ cup pasta sauce
3 ounces chicken breast
1½ cups steamed broccoli
1½ tablespoons olive oil

Total: Carbohydrates (67 grams) + Fat (29 grams) + Protein (38 grams) + 12 grams fiber

Notice: Compared to the USDA pasta meal example, this dish has half the amount of pasta; broccoli fills nearly half the plate; the meat portion is increased; additional healthy fat is included.

We emphasize that whole grains and starchy vegetables can be included in a healthy diet, but they should be underemphasized compared to the amount of vegetables on your plate. For many Americans, the USDA model has contributed to a whole array of metabolic disorders due to its high amount of carbohydrates and underemphasis of fats. Add in the food industry, which has made cheap, refined carbohydrates easily accessible, and it is no surprise that many Americans are dealing with obesity and diabetes. By filling half your plate with non-starchy vegetables, you are decreasing the real estate available for less nutrient-dense carbs. By emphasizing healthy fat with every meal, you are providing your taste buds as well as your brain with a sense of satiety. By including a healthy portion size of protein on your plate, you ensure slow, sustaining energy between mealtimes.

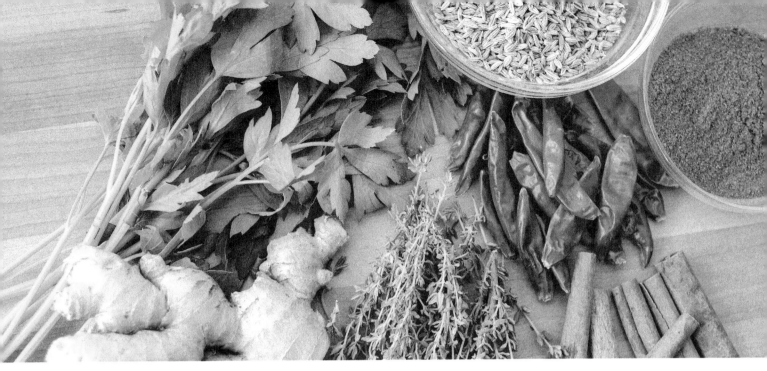

CHAPTER SEVEN

Strategies For Healthy Digestion

I have relaxed around food in general and preparing whole foods—it takes time and it's worth it to eat food I know is good for me and my family. This is a big deal for me. Before this class, I was always worried about weight management. My time with this project has freed me from this negative preoccupation.

—Patricia, FAME series, Charlee's Kitchen

WHERE DOES DIGESTION START? IN THE MOUTH? IN THE STOMACH? ACTUALLY, THE DIGESTIVE PROCESS STARTS IN THE BRAIN! Consider the following visualization exercise:

Sit with closed eyes. Take a few deep breaths. Now, imagine that there is a lemon sitting on a table. Take a knife and slice the lemon. Take half of the lemon and squeeze it into a glass. Pick up the glass and take a sip of the fresh squeezed lemon juice.

How do you feel? Did you notice any changes in your body?

Most people will begin to salivate or feel their mouths pucker with just the thought of the lemon juice. Salivation indicates that the mouth has secreted enzymes that begin the digestive process. Thus, just by imagining food in the mind, your body has started physiological processes to break down food!

Ever hear the phrase, "You are what you eat?" It is more accurate to say, "You are what you eat, digest, absorb, and eliminate." Digestion is a complex process that turns the food we eat into usable energy and nutrients for the body. Digestion is also very heavily influenced by the state of mind or environment we are in while eating. Consider if you have ever eaten food or a meal in the following environments:

Driving a car?
Talking on the phone?
Working at your desk?
Surfing the internet on your computer, tablet, or smartphone?
Reading a book or newspaper?
During a stressful discussion?
Watching TV?
When in a hurry?

All of the above activities have the potential to affect your digestion in a negative way. To understand this more, let's look at the way our nervous system directly influences digestion.

The Nervous System

Generally speaking, the nervous system responds to our environment or thoughts in two distinct ways: the **parasympathetic** and the **sympathetic** systems.

The Sympathetic State

The **sympathetic state** is also known as *fight or flight*. The classic example of being in a sympathetic state is the concept of being chased by a bear. When running from a bear, the sympathetic state allows the body to run faster and hit harder. Currently, people don't usually find themselves running from a bear very often. But, we can equate these physiologic changes to *any* stressful situation in which we might find ourselves.

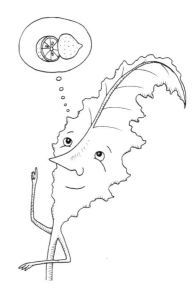

Sit with closed eyes.
Take a few deep breaths.
Now, imagine that there is a lemon sitting on a table.
Take a knife and slice the lemon. Take half of the lemon and squeeze it into a glass.
Pick up the glass and take a sip of the fresh squeezed lemon juice. How do you feel?
Did you notice any changes in your body?

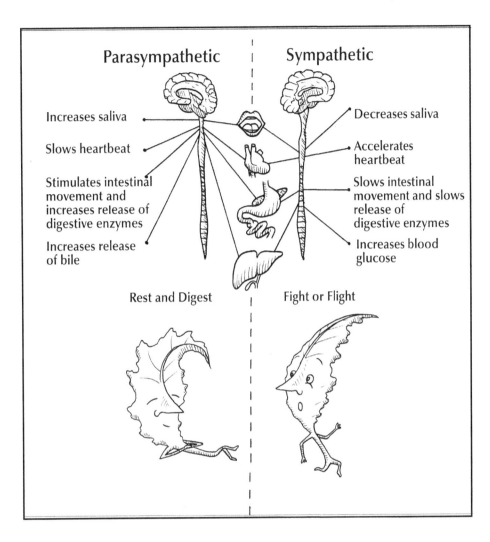

The diagram above shows some of the effects on the body when in a sympathetic state. Notice what happens to the digestive process when in this state. All of the digestive processes are slowed or stopped, including saliva flow, digestive enzyme secretion, and intestinal contractions to move the food along. While the sympathetic nervous system is a natural and necessary part of our human reaction, our society tends to create the state of stress—more often than not—including when we are eating meals. Rushing to work and school, balancing hectic schedules, dealing with financial stress, and the constant bombardment of negative news and media: all of these factors contribute to a chronic sympathetic state of mind.

The Parasympathetic State

The **parasympathetic state** is known as ***rest and digest.*** In a calm, low-stress environment with limited stimulation, the body will be in a parasympathetic state. Notice what happens with digestion when in a parasympathetic state: saliva and digestive enzymes are secreted, and the smooth intestinal muscles move the food along for optimal digestion and absorption. Digestion will improve, including a decrease in minor digestive complaints, such as gas and bloating, that often accompany rushed eating. In a restful state, we are also more likely to notice when we feel full, decreasing the chance of overeating. While most people lead busy lives and often find themselves eating in stressful situations, there are simple ways to create an environment for eating that will help stimulate the *rest and digest* response.

Strategies For Healthy Digestion

- Turn off all electronic devices, including TV's, phones, tablets, and computers during meals.

- Take the time to put the food on a plate and find a comfortable space to eat. Sit down while eating. If eating at work, find an area to eat other than at the desk.

- Take ten deep, slow belly breaths before beginning to eat. This is a powerful and simple way to create a parasympathetic state. It is also a good time to acknowledge and give thanks for where the food came from and who prepared it.

- Connect with your food. If preparing the meals, smell the food, which will start the digestive process. Take the time to actually look at the meal before eating and to admire its colors and presentation.

- Put down the fork between bites and focus on chewing the food. This is an easy and often overlooked way to improve digestion. Aim to chew each bite until the food is near liquid in the mouth.

In a calm, low-stress environment with limited stimulation, the body will be in a parasympathetic state. Notice what happens with digestion when in a parasympathetic state: saliva and digestive enzymes are secreted, and the smooth intestinal muscles move the food along for optimal digestion and absorption. Digestion will improve, including a decrease in minor digestive complaints, such as gas and bloating, that often accompany rushed eating.

Practice mindful eating. Avoid multi-tasking, just eat. Savor the flavor, texture, and taste of your food. Observe how you feel before, during, and after the meal.

Connect with your food. If preparing the meals, smell the food, which will start the digestive process. Take the time to actually look at the meal before eating and admire its colors and presentation.

- Limit fluid intake during meals. Drink small amounts of water if thirsty. Aim to drink water between meals to avoid being excessively thirsty during meals.

- Eat slowly and stop eating before feeling completely full. If you are eating fast, or are distracted while eating, there is the potential to overeat.

- Practice mindful eating. Avoid multi-tasking; just eat. Savor the flavor, texture, and taste of your food. Observe how you feel before, during, and after the meal.

- Experiment and add different spices, herbs, and other foods to meals that aid in digestion, such as fennel, ginger, cinnamon, lemon, apple cider vinegar, cayenne or black pepper. Apple cider vinegar can lower post-meal blood sugar levels, slow carbohydrate absorption, and improve satiety![1] Add 1 to 2 tablespoons to the meal or drink 1 to 2 teaspoons in a small glass of water 15 minutes before meals. Our recipe section lists delicious dressings that include healthy oils with apple cider vinegar to reap these benefits.

These digestive strategies are often effective at dealing with *minor* digestive complaints such as gas, bloating, and heartburn that are the result of eating in a sympathetic state. However, there are many other factors that affect digestion, absorption, and elimination. Examples are the quality of intestinal bacteria, food sensitivities and allergies, underlying infections, medications, and chronic inflammation from a poor Standard American Diet and lifestyle. We further explore healthy intestinal bacteria because they are so essential to optimal digestion.

Healthy Bacteria: The Role Of Probiotics

Gut flora, specifically healthy bacteria, is a key component of the immune system. Billions of bacteria line the length of the digestive tract, maintaining a layer of protection so that more harmful bacteria cannot invade the digestive tract and make us sick. Healthy bacteria support digestion, absorption of nutrients, elimination of toxins, regular bowel movements, and the balance of hormones and inflammation.[2,3,4,5,6,7]

Thus, it is important that healthy bacteria are replenished and supported regularly. Traditionally, this was achieved by eating fermented foods, a great source of probiotics, on a *daily* basis. Currently, few Americans eat any fermented foods. In addition, stress, a diet low in fiber and high in refined carbohydrates, and antibiotics create imbalance in healthy gut bacteria levels. Antibiotics kill pathogenic (harmful) bacteria, but they also kill healthy bacteria and allow susceptibility for overgrowth of other harmful bacteria and yeast.

Tips to Support Healthy Bacteria

Eat foods high in soluble fiber, such as fruits, vegetables, whole grains, and beans, which help to support the growth and maintenance of healthy bacteria in the gut. Foods like Jerusalem artichokes, jicama, and chicory root are high in *inulin*, a type of fiber and food source for gut bacteria.

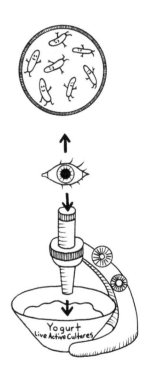

On a food label, the presence of healthy bacteria would be indicated by the term *live active cultures*. This label is not regulated and will not confirm the number or quality of organisms. The following fermented foods are rich in healthy bacteria:

dairy, goat, sheep, or coconut yogurt and kefir

kombucha

kimchi

fermented soy foods: tempeh, miso, natto, tamari

pickles and sauerkraut (Traditionally, pickles and sauerkraut were fermented. Most commercial brands today are not fermented; they are only made with vinegar. Check health food stores or local farmers' markets and look for the term *live active cultures*.)

Look for Live, Active Yogurt!

A further note about yogurt: all conventional milk is pasteurized, which is a high-heat process that kills bacteria, both friendly and harmful. To make yogurt, live cultures (commonly, *Lactobacillus sp.* and *Streptococcus thermophilus*) are added to ferment the pasteurized milk. However, oftentimes, a second heat process is used to treat the

To make yogurt, live cultures (commonly, Lactobacillus sp. and Streptococcus thermophilus) are added to ferment the pasteurized milk. However, oftentimes, a second heat process is used to treat the yogurt, killing most of the live cultures. Be sure to read the food label to find the brands that maintain live active cultures.

yogurt, killing most of the live cultures. Be sure to read the food label to find the brands that maintain *live active cultures.*

The amount of healthy bacteria can vary naturally in a fermented food. In general, the best option is to eat a variety of fermented foods. Naturopathic doctors often recommend supplementing with a high quality probiotic which provides specific strains and amounts of healthy bacteria for diets that are lacking daily sources of fermented food. A probiotic supplement can be used to prevent and treat specific conditions including diarrhea, inflammatory bowel disease, atopic diseases—including eczema and allergies—vaginitis, and bladder infections. A probiotic supplement can also be used for generalized immune support to prevent viral and bacterial infections.[8]

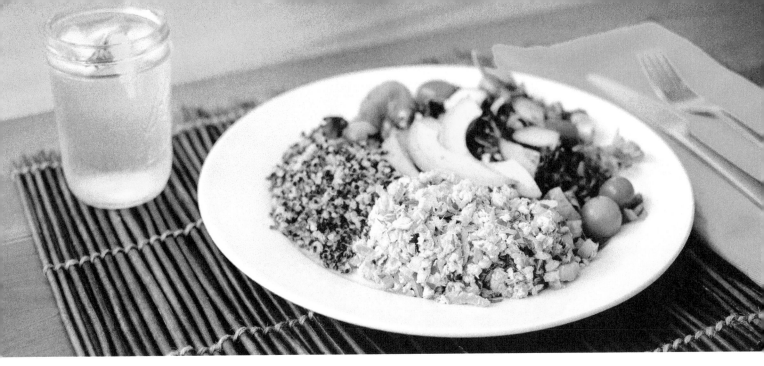

CHAPTER EIGHT

Balancing Blood Sugar

HERE IS A STORY OF SOMEONE TO WHOM YOU CAN PROBABLY RELATE. SARA IS A 39-YEAR-OLD FULL-TIME WORKING WOMAN. She loves her office job in marketing, even though it requires long hours and can be stressful to meet multiple deadlines. Sara begins her day by peeling herself out of bed, not feeling rested from the night before. She has to hurry out the door to get to work on time, but she does find time to make her daily stop at the local coffee shop for a triple skinny vanilla latte and a scone. Sara has become dependent on this ritual, for the energy from the caffeine, but also the social contact. Around 10:30 a.m., after a few hours of work, Sara feels tired, irritable, and starved. She usually has a granola bar in her desk to hold her over until lunch. After sitting behind a desk all morning, Sara is excited for lunch and usually walks to her building's cafeteria to grab a piece of pizza, side salad, and a diet soda. She finds her energy picks up at the lunch break. After returning to work, Sara anticipates her daily 3 p.m. energy crash and grabs an energy drink from the office kitchen to pull her through until 5 p.m. Sara looks forward to a glass or two of wine with girlfriends at the end of a packed workday. She heads home and throws a pasta dinner in the microwave while sitting down to enjoy some TV before bedtime.

Sara would say she is a relatively happy, positive person, but she would love to have more energy during the day, to sleep more deeply at night, and to lose about 10 to 15 pounds. She admits to low motivation regarding increasing daily physical activity, since she devotes most of her energy to work and friends. Sara's story is a typical example of someone eating the Standard American Diet, which is low in nutrients and high in calories (and caffeine in her case). Sara will likely be able to continue this routine for a few years before she becomes frustrated with her low energy, has some nagging health symptoms, and seeks medical advice. Sara needs some practical support to balance her blood sugar on a daily basis.

The body works very hard to maintain blood sugar (glucose) levels within a tight range. If the level goes too low, it is called hypoglycemia. This often happens when we skip meals during the day or, ironically, as a consequence of feasting on sweets. Common symptoms of hypoglycemia include fatigue, irritability, foggy thinking, dizziness, and in extreme cases, fainting and loss of consciousness.

On the other hand, the body can experience hyperglycemia, or elevated blood sugar levels, for long periods of time (we're talking days, months, and years) without showing any noticeable symptoms. This is another kind of danger: silently elevated blood sugar can put one at risk for metabolic syndrome, diabetes, and heart disease—currently the number **one** cause of death for both men and women in the United States.

Body mass is impacted by blood sugar regulation. It is difficult to maintain a healthy weight or to maintain weight loss when the body is put through extended periods of **either** low or high blood sugar.

While food choice is a central piece of balancing blood sugar, your body's hormones also strongly influence blood sugar balance. Understanding basic hormone functions in the body will encourage behavioral strategies and changes which will in turn improve hormone function.

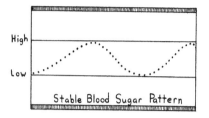

Stable Blood Sugar Pattern

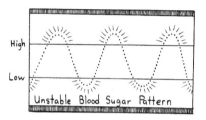

Unstable Blood Sugar Pattern

The body works very hard to maintain a tight range of blood sugar level (blood glucose). If the level goes too low, it is called hypoglycemia. This often happens when we skip meals during the day or, ironically, as a consequence of feasting on sweets. Common symptoms of hypoglycemia include fatigue, irritability, foggy thinking, dizziness, and in extreme cases, fainting and loss of consciousness.

Hormones 101

Insulin

The pancreas secretes insulin when blood sugar rises following a meal. Refined and simple carbohydrates are especially effective at stimulating insulin. When the body is balanced, insulin unlocks the door of the cells for glucose to enter. When the body is imbalanced by poor dietary choices, stress, or medical conditions such as diabetes or metabolic syndrome, the cells of the body become resistant to insulin's activity. This means that insulin is at the cell to unlock its door, but it does not open, leaving both insulin and glucose in the blood. This is called insulin resistance. This condition has some seriously risky consequences, including increased risk for prediabetes and ultimately diabetes. Additionally, excess insulin promotes belly fat.

Glucagon

In its wisdom, the body has a buddy hormone to counterbalance insulin. In times of fasting or low blood sugar, glucagon works to release stored glucose from the liver, making it available in the blood stream for cell use. The insulin-glucagon relationship represents the body's ability to maintain blood sugar balance quite well even under an episode of fasting or high caloric feasting. If these episodes of excess or deficient caloric intake occur chronically over years, this self-regulating system begins to show signs of deterioration.

Cortisol

Also known as *the stress hormone*, cortisol is secreted by the adrenal glands, which are located above each of the kidneys. Cortisol, when released during times of stress (whether physical, mental or emotional), will cause a rise in blood sugar, which ultimately leads to an insulin response. Cortisol also blunts the effects of insulin on the cell doors, increasing risk of insulin resistance. The effect of chronic stress on insulin resistance ultimately leads to chronic blood sugar dysregulation and weight gain, especially around the midsection.

Hormones are impacted by both behavior and lifestyle choices

When the body is imbalanced by poor dietary choices, stress, or medical conditions such as diabetes or metabolic syndrome, the cells of the body become resistant to insulin's activity. This means that insulin is at the cell to unlock its door, but it does not open, leaving both insulin and glucose in the blood. This is called insulin resistance.

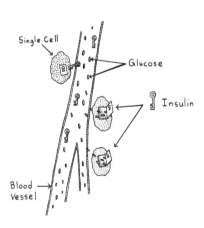

as well as by the foods you eat. Consider the following strategies to support balanced hormones and blood sugar.

Essential Strategies To Balance Blood Sugar

1. *Do NOT skip breakfast*

Following a nighttime of fasting, breakfast is the most important meal of the day and jump-starts your metabolism. It may sound cliché, but truly, don't skip breakfast. Refer to Chapter Ten, **Benefits of Breakfast**, for more information about the importance of this meal.

2. *Be cautious about skipping other meals*

Skipping meals is ***stressful***, especially in today's busy, fast-paced lifestyle. Most people respond best to three meals a day. Optimally, our bodies are built to sustain extended periods of fasting, whether four to five hours between meals or a twelve hour nightly fast. The truth is that each body is different, and life circumstances will dictate an individual's optimal meal schedule.

3. *Protein, Fat, and Fiber—The PFFs*

Slow fuels help to support healthy blood sugar levels. Don't skip out on healthy sources of protein, fat, or fiber at every meal. Remember, aim for 35 to 50 grams of fiber daily, which means including 10 to 20 grams per meal, depending upon how often one is eating throughout the day. Fiber, in particular, will help to regulate the body's insulin response by slowing digestion and absorption of the dietary carbohydrates or sugars that have been consumed.

4. *Do NOT avoid fat*

The key is to eat healthy fats.

5. *Water, water, water!*

It is not uncommon to think you are hungry when you are actually thirsty due to dehydration. And, with easy access to calorie-rich drinks, like fruit juice, energy drinks, and flavored *water* drinks, it is easy to see how quick, simple calories can be brought into the daily diet when one is not staying adequately hydrated with pure water. A good guideline is to drink half your body weight (in pounds) in

Most people respond best to three meals a day. Optimally, our bodies are built to sustain extended periods of fasting, whether four to five hours between meals or a twelve hour nightly fast. The truth is that each body is different, and life circumstances will dictate an individual's optimal meal schedule.

ounces of water daily. If you have been diagnosed with heart or kidney disease, check with your doctor before significantly increasing water intake due to the added stress on those organs.

6. *Problem carbohydrates*

Avoid or limit common carbs that contribute to many health problems:

- common table sugar, honey, maple syrup, and any other added sweeteners consumed in excess (explored further in Chapter Nine, **Exploring Sweeteners**);

- refined grains like white pasta, white bread, white rice;

- fructose from fruit juices and foods containing high-fructose corn syrup;

- cookies, candy, chips;

- pastries;

- soda pop, fruit juice, and energy drinks;

- alcoholic beverages in excess.

Consuming alcohol in moderation can provide health benefits such as reduced risk of heart disease and diabetes.[1,2,3] The key is to understand the role of moderation as well as your personal health history. It is essential to understand what moderate intake means: an average of one to two drinks per day for men and one drink per day for women.

A drink is defined as 12 ounces of beer, 4 ounces of wine, 1.5 ounces of 80-proof spirits, or 1 ounce of 100-proof spirits. While red wine adds some special benefits to your heart and your brain due to phytonutrients, such as the antioxidant resveratrol, any form of alcohol can contribute to raising your protective cholesterol, HDL.[4,5] Contrary to popular belief, drinking alcohol does not cause a rise in blood sugar. Moderate alcohol consumption actually lowers one's risk of developing Type II diabetes. One proposed mechanism is that alcohol increases insulin sensitivity, allowing for more effective carbohydrate utilization by the

A good guideline is to drink half your body weight (in pounds) in ounces of water daily.

If you have been diagnosed with heart or kidney disease, check with your doctor before significantly increasing water intake due to the added stress on those organs.

cells.[6,7,8] This may be one of the benefits of choosing to drink a glass of wine with a carbohydrate-rich meal. Drinking wine in particular may have additional benefits by slowing gastric emptying and thereby the rate at which the glucose level rises in the blood following a meal.[9] On the flip side, the body will preferentially choose to burn calories from alcohol over other calories consumed in a meal from fats, carbs, and proteins. This means that alcohol does contribute to added calories in the diet and will contribute to weight gain if its impact on total daily caloric intake is not taken into consideration.

The serving size, type of alcohol and type of mixer consumed are important considerations in the context of added calories. Choose mixers wisely, as many are loaded with added sweeteners. Unlike tonic water, club soda does not contain added sweeteners. See Table 8.1 to compare the serving size, alcohol content, and calories of common alcoholic beverages.

The health benefits of alcohol must be weighed against the known dangers of excessive drinking, including alcoholism, high blood pressure, obesity, fatty liver disease, cancer (including liver cancer, breast cancer in women, colon cancer in men, and oral cancers), suicide and accidents.[10]

Because of these dangers and the fact that alcohol is not an essential part of a well balanced diet, we don't recommend starting to drink if you don't already. However, if you do enjoy a daily drink, consider choosing red wine and know that you are gaining some heart-healthy benefits.

Contrary to popular belief, drinking alcohol does not cause a rise in blood sugar. Light to moderate alcohol consumption actually lowers one's risk of developing Type II diabetes. One proposed mechanism is that alcohol increases insulin sensitivity, allowing for more effective carbohydrate utilization by cells. This may be one of the benefits of choosing to drink a glass of wine with a carbohydrate-rich meal.

Table 8.1 Nutrition Values for Alcoholic Beverages and Mixes

Beverage	Serving Size (ounces)	Alcohol Content (grams)	Carbohydrates (grams)	Calories
Regular beer	12	13	13	150
Distilled spirits, 80-proof (gin, rum, vodka, whiskey, scotch)	1.5	14	Trace	100
White wine	4	11	Trace	80
Red wine	4	12	2	85
Wine cooler	12	13	30	215
Champagne	4	12	4	100

7. *Stress management*

Practice stress management techniques daily, such as deep breathing, meditation, yoga, walking outside, gentle exercise, praying or saying words of gratitude, talking with a trusted friend, or playing with a pet. Remember that there will always be stress in your life. This is **normal**. Being mindful of your stress, both the good kind and the bad kind, is part of a stress management plan. The activities listed above are time-tested lifestyle choices that help bodies and minds adapt to a stressful world.

8. *Move every day*

For at least 30 minutes, ideally 60 to 90 minutes, do something you enjoy. Daily movement is non-negotiable for those most at risk for pre-diabetes or those who have entered the realm of Metabolic Syndrome (see following page). Exercise will stimulate and build muscles that will improve insulin sensitivity not only during exercise, but all day long! Movement does not have to mean a trip to the gym. You can simply dance at home, walk 10,000 steps (approximately 5 miles) throughout the day, or start walking the stairs at your workplace before, during, and after the workday. Be active throughout the day and avoid sitting for long periods of time. Interrupt every sixty minutes of sitting with five minutes of stretching or walking.

9. Sleep

Maintaining a healthy sleep and wake cycle is essential to health and to maintaining a healthy weight. Hormone balance depends on establishing a sleep routine. Aim to be in bed before midnight and to sleep for at least eight hours nightly. Sleep in a very dark room.

Making lifestyle changes takes time and commitment, as well as constant inspiration and motivation. Surround yourself with positive people who will support you along the way.

Metabolic Syndrome

Are you on your way to diabetes or heart disease and don't know it? You may be if you find yourself dealing with the following:

- struggling with weight gain despite sustained efforts to lose weight
- excessive belly fat
- moving very little in your daily life
- a history of high blood pressure or high cholesterol
- eating a Standard American Diet (SAD)

Metabolic Syndrome is a state of hormone imbalance in the body involving insulin, glucagon and cortisol. Metabolic syndrome may be putting you in harm's way years before the development of heart disease or diabetes.

This syndrome is considered to be a cluster of common abnormalities, including insulin resistance, impaired glucose tolerance, abdominal obesity, reduced HDL-cholesterol levels, elevated triglycerides, and hypertension.

Those who are overweight or obese are at increased risk, especially those that carry extra pounds around the middle of their body or waist.

Insulin resistance certainly plays a key role in the creation of this syndrome.

The strongest risk factors for the development of this metabolic syndrome are obesity, a highly processed diet with poor quality fats, low fiber intake, and a lack of physical activity.

Type II Diabetes Mellitus Defined

Diabetes Mellitus is characterized by fasting hyperglycemia (elevated blood glucose) and glycosuria (spilling of excess glucose in the urine). Diabetes is a chronic disease that requires strict management and often multiple treatments, including dietary and lifestyle changes, nutritional supplements and medication. This is not to say that the symptoms and health consequences of diabetes cannot be successfully managed, but it can be a tough road that requires a lifetime commitment.

What To Know About Diabetes

Adult onset or Type II diabetes results from abnormal pancreas function caused by insulin resistance in the cells. Insulin resistance is when the cells stop responding to insulin, thus keeping glucose from entering the cells, resulting in high amounts of glucose in the blood. As long as there is too much glucose in the blood and not enough in the cells, the pancreas will continue to produce insulin, eventually wearing it out and causing it to stop producing sufficient insulin. The build-up of glucose in the blood can result in very serious complications.

Over time, the excess blood sugar deposits in the smallest blood vessels (the capillaries), resulting in increased risk for atherosclerosis (heart disease), nephropathy (kidney disease), retinopathy (eye disease), and neuropathy (nerve disease). Excess blood sugar also causes an increased risk of infections due to depressed immunity and poor wound healing.

Symptoms a person with diabetes may experience include polydipsia (increased thirst), polyuria (increased frequency of urination), fatigue, and weight loss. Some people have diabetes and are not experiencing *any* symptoms at all. While the body is quick to react to significantly low blood sugar levels, years can pass before one realizes the consequences of unmanaged hyperglycemia.

Diabetes management requires regular blood glucose monitoring to measure the impact of different foods and activities on blood sugar levels. Exercise is key, as are diet, sleep, stress management, and very likely natural or pharmaceutical medication. Diagnosis can be determined by a visit to your primary care provider, who will look for:

Elevation of fasting blood sugar above 126 mg/dl on two separate blood tests or elevation of non-fasting blood sugar above 200 mg/dl.

Hemoglobin A1c (HbA1c) of 6.5% or higher. HbA1c is a blood test that measures average blood sugar levels over three months.

Pre-diabetes is a fasting blood sugar over 100 mg/dl or a HbA1c between 5.7% and 6.4%.

Table 8.2 Important Nutrients and Their Food Sources for Diabetes

Nutrient	Function	Food Sources
Vitamin C	Influences collagen production, wound healing, immune function, and serves as a potent antioxidant.	Broccoli, bell peppers, citrus fruit, Brussels sprouts, strawberries
Vitamin D	Immune-stimulating and cardio-protective properties. Reduces insulin resistance.[11]	Fish and cod liver oil, dairy from pasture-raised cows and goats, mushrooms, sardines, and *sunshine—the best non-food source*
Zinc	Influences synthesis, storage and release of insulin. Supports healthy immune response. Aids in wound healing.	Oysters, red meat, poultry, legumes, nuts, pumpkin seeds
Chromium	Improves insulin sensitivity.[12]	Broccoli, tomatoes, romaine lettuce, green beans, whole grains (bran), brewer's yeast, black pepper
Omega-3 Fatty Acids	Incorporated into cell membranes and promote anti-inflammatory chemical messengers in the body.	Fish and cod liver oil, pasture-raised meat, poultry and eggs, wild game, ground flaxseed, chia seeds, walnuts
Antioxidants	Increases capillary integrity and improves vascular tone.	Blueberries, bilberries, and all brightly colored fruits and vegetables

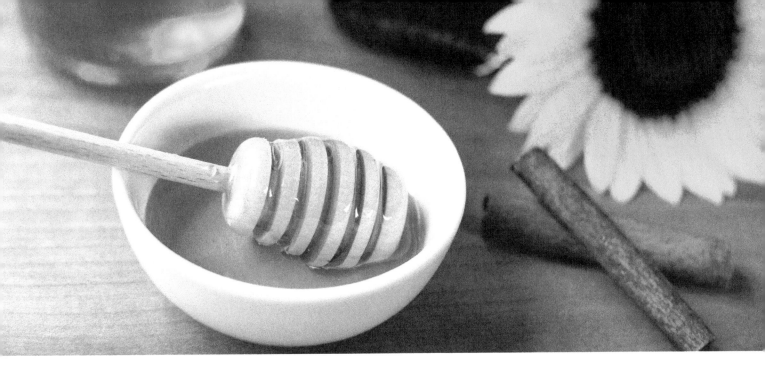

Chapter Nine

Exploring Sweeteners

In today's food supply, Americans can readily access cheap, abundant sources of added sugar. With easy access and a built-in desire for sugar, it is no wonder that we are over-consuming cheap sweet treats. Tragically, the excess consumption of sugar is contributing to obesity, heart disease, diabetes, dental cavities, decreased immune function, and other metabolic disorders.

Added sugar in food or drinks contributes to the intake of discretionary calories, or those calories that are not essential to provide energy or nutrients for the body. The body doesn't *need* added sugar in the diet, so aiming to eliminate added sugar on a daily basis and saving it for rare occasions is ideal. *Added sugar* does not refer to natural sugars found in whole foods and unprocessed whole fruit, vegetables, and dairy. Unfortunately, food labels do not currently identify whether the grams of sugar are from naturally occurring or added sugars, nor do they indicate the percent daily value (%DV). Recently, in 2014 and 2015, the FDA proposed label changes to more accurately reflect the source of sugar and the contribution to daily caloric intake. However, once these new guidelines are accepted, it can still take years for food labels to reflect the changes. *Therefore, it is critical to read the ingredient list, to estimate the amount of added versus natural sugar, and to know the sources of added sugar in foods and beverages.*

Read the *ingredients list* to see if added sugar or sweeteners are a part of the food or drink. It is not as easy as simply looking for the word *sugar*. Here are some additional ingredients found on labels and indicating that a form of sweetener has been added.

INGREDIENTS: AGAVE, BROWN SUGAR, CANE CRYSTALS, CANE JUICE, CANE SUGAR, CORN SWEETENER, CORN SYRUP, CRYSTALLINE FRUCTOSE, DEXTROSE, EVAPORATED CANE JUICE, FRUCTOSE, FRUIT JUICE CONCENTRATES, GLUCOSE, HIGH-FRUCTOSE CORN SYRUP, HONEY, INVERT SUGAR, LACTOSE, MALTOSE, MALT SYRUP, MOLASSES, RAW SUGAR, SUCROSE, SUGAR, SYRUP

The American Heart Association recommends that women consume less than six teaspoons of added sugar or sweeteners a day and that men consume less than nine teaspoons of added sugar or sweeteners a day.

Since most people are consuming excessive amounts, it is helpful to have a reference point for an upper limit of added sugar intake. The American Heart Association (AHA) recommends that women consume less than *six teaspoons* of added sugar or sweeteners a day and that men consume less than *nine teaspoons* of added sugar or sweeteners a day.

While teaspoons are a great visual when measuring sugar at home, food labels present sugar in grams and calories. The AHA recommendations can be translated into the following equations:

6 teaspoons = 24 grams of sugar= 90 calories
9 teaspoons = 36 grams =135 calories

To simplify further, remember this basic equation:

1 teaspoon = 4 grams = 15 calories

A helpful reference is a package of sugar typically found at a restaurant which contains 4 grams or 15 calories or 1 teaspoon of sugar.

As for teenagers, the amount of added sugar consumed daily is

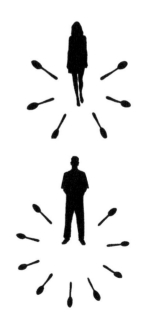

staggering. The National Health and Nutrition Examination Survey (NHANES) of 2,157 teenagers (ages 12 to 18) found the average daily consumption of added sugars was 119 grams (or 28.3 teaspoons), accounting for 21.4% of their total calories.[1] Sweetened beverages have been identified as the main culprit to this shocking finding. While the obvious prevalence of childhood obesity in our country has many contributing factors, easy access to and high consumption of sweetened beverages by kids and teens is one of the most significant. Daily caloric intake in children and teens is dependent on individual needs and physical activity level. However, aiming for *less* than 10% of daily caloric intake from added sweeteners is a starting place. Because children vary widely in their caloric need based on size, development, and growth rate, this can be a challenging number to calculate. The less added sugar the better, and aiming for less than 5 teaspoons a day is a healthy start, especially when considering teenagers are getting close to 30 teaspoons of added sweeteners daily.

To make sense of the upper limit recommendation when looking at a food label, see the following examples. You will be shocked at how much added sweetener is in commonly consumed beverages!

Coca-Cola ®
   (12 ounces): 39 grams sugar (almost 10 teaspoons)
Mountain Dew ®
   (20 ounces): 77 grams sugar (19¼ teaspoons)
Blue Sky ® Natural Soda, Cherry Vanilla Cream
   (12 ounces): 46 grams sugar (11½ teaspoons)
Vitaminwater™ Orange-Orange
   (20 ounces): 32.5 grams sugar (8 teaspoons)
Washington Natural Apple Juice ®
   (16 ounces): 56 grams sugar (14 teaspoons)

Sweetened beverages can significantly add to daily caloric intake and add little to healthy nutrition in the daily diet. It is common to be distracted by the words *natural* or *organic* on a beverage label and to assume incorrectly that it is lower in added sugar. Popular

Sweetened beverages **can significantly add** *to daily caloric intake and add little to healthy nutrition in the daily diet. It is common to be distracted by the words* **natural** *or* **organic** *on a beverage label and to assume incorrectly that it is lower in added sugar. Popular vitamin drinks may have added some extra vitamins, but generally, one of these drinks will put most people above the upper limit of added sugar for the day.*

vitamin drinks may have added some extra vitamins, but generally, one of these drinks will put most people above the upper limit of added sugar for the day. 100% fruit juice can provide some important vitamins and antioxidants; however, with the loss of the fiber from the whole fruit, the juice becomes an added sugar, and one that is very high in fructose. As for soda and energy drinks, the negative effects of the sugar and caffeine will exceed any nutritional benefit of added supplemental vitamins and minerals.

The Centers for Disease Control (CDC) reports that Americans have significantly increased their soda intake in the last 30 years.[2] In the past, soda bottles were much smaller and not consumed on a regular basis due to access and cost. Now, soda comes in super sizes and with free refills. With vending machines everywhere, it is easy to create a society of soda drinkers.

While the obvious prevalence of childhood obesity in our country has many contributing factors, easy access to and high consumption of sweetened beverages by kids and teens is one of the most significant.

Reasons To Avoid Soda

- Give the liver a break. Most sodas contain high-fructose corn syrup, which is metabolized in part by the liver and leads, in excess, to fatty changes in the liver as well as elevated triglycerides.[3] Corn syrup sweeteners are often genetically modified. They also contain a high percentage of glucose, leading to a high insulin spike following consumption.

- Drinking soda erodes and darkens teeth.[4]

- Drinking soda increases the risk of osteoporosis. This is due to the phosphoric acid in the soda, which inhibits calcium absorption. Children and adolescents who drink soda are also at risk.[5,6]

- Soda increases the risk of weight gain and development of Type II diabetes.[7]

- Soda consumption distracts people from good hydration. Water is often neglected in place of soda.

- Many sodas contain artificial sweeteners, flavorings, colorings, and added caffeine.

Most sodas contain high-fructose corn syrup, which is metabolized in part by the liver and leads, in excess, to fatty changes in the liver as well as elevated triglycerides. Remember that corn syrup sweeteners are often genetically modified. They also contain a high percentage of glucose, leading to a big insulin spike following consumption.

Challenge yourself to go an entire week without any sodas or sugared beverages. Notice if you drink more water, if sugar cravings are less, or if there are other physical or mental changes without soda.

Alternative Drinks To Soda:

herbal teas, such as mint or chamomile, served iced or hot;

water with cucumber, mint, or rosemary;

water with a squeeze of lemon, lime, or orange;

sparkling or mineral water with lemon, lime, orange, or berries;

pure water.

For those who are currently fruit juice drinkers, begin by diluting your juice by adding 60 to 75% of water to pure fruit juice. For instance, start by mixing 1/3 cup juice with 2/3 cup water.

Natural Versus Added Sugar

Consider the example of yogurt. This is a common food that contains both naturally occurring sugars (primarily lactose) and may also contain added sugars (cane sugar or high-fructose corn syrup). A container of plain, unsweetened yogurt will often show 11 grams of sugar on the label. The ingredient list will indicate that no added sugar is included. This means that the 11 grams of sugar are from naturally occurring milk sugars and not considered *added sugar* in the diet.

A flavored container of yogurt will often contain up to 30 to 35 grams of sugar. One can make a good assumption that compared to plain yogurt, it is likely that up to 19 to 24 grams of sweeteners has been added to the flavored yogurt, or approximately 5 to 6 teaspoons of sweeteners. It is only by reading the ingredient list that the consumer can determine if there are added sweeteners. Because flavored yogurts are such a big source of added sweeteners, we suggest having plain yogurt and adding your own chopped fruits and nuts and a small amount (1 teaspoon or less) of honey or maple syrup, if needed.

See the yogurt labels below and compare the grams of sugar per serving in the ingredient listing.

Nutrition Facts	
Serving Size 8oz. (227g)	
Servings Per Container 1	
Amount Per Serving	
Calories 149 Calories from Fat 72	
	% Daily Value*
Total Fat 7.96g	12%
Saturated Fat 5.14g	26%
Trans Fat 0g	0%
Polyunsaturated Fat 0g	0%
Monounsaturated Fat 0g	0%
Cholesterol 31.85mg	11%
Sodium 112.7mg	5%
Total Carbohydrate 11.42g	4%
Dietary Fiber 0g	0%
Sugars 11.42g	
Protein 8.5g	
Vitamin A 5% • Vitamin C 2%	
Calcium 30% • Iron 1%	

INGREDIENTS: CULTURED PASTEURIZED MILK, LIVE AND ACTIVE CULTURES: S. THERMOPHILUS, L. ACIDOPHILUS.

Nutrition Facts	
Serving Size 8oz. (227g)	
Servings Per Container 1	
Amount Per Serving	
Calories 238 Calories from Fat 29	
	% Daily Value*
Total Fat 3.2g	5%
Saturated Fat 2.06g	10%
Trans Fat 0g	0%
Polyunsaturated Fat 0g	0%
Monounsaturated Fat 0g	0%
Cholesterol 13.62mg	5%
Sodium 147.55mg	6%
Total Carbohydrate 42.22g	14%
Dietary Fiber 0g	0%
Sugars 33g	
Protein 11.03g	
Vitamin A 3% • Vitamin C 3%	
Calcium 38% • Iron 1%	

INGREDIENTS: CULTURED PASTEURIZED MILK, EVAPORATED CANE JUICE, BLUEBERRIES, NATURAL VANILLA FLAVOR, LOCUST BEAN GUM, PECTIN, LIVE AND ACTIVE CULTURES: S. THERMOPHILUS, L. ACIDOPHILUS.

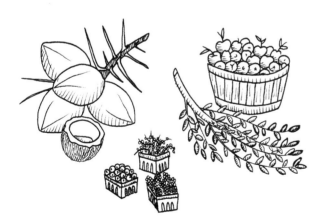

Why Care About Added Sugar In The Diet?

Optimizing Blood Sugar Control

As discussed in the previous chapter, the human body requires blood sugar to be maintained in a very narrow range to preserve balance, or homeostasis, in the body. Glucose is the preferred source of energy for the entire body, especially the brain.

Recall that the main responsibility of insulin is to manage blood sugar levels in the body. Insulin allows blood glucose to enter the cells to provide essential fuel. The stimulus for insulin secretion by the pancreas is high blood glucose, which occurs following a meal or a calorie-rich beverage. A diet high in sugar and refined carbohydrates can cause more severe fluctuations of glucose and insulin, leading to insulin resistance.

Some basic biochemistry can help us understand why *too much sugar in any form can be detrimental*. Table sugar is known as sucrose, a disaccharide, and is composed of two monosaccharides, 50% glucose and 50% fructose. Fructose does not increase insulin like glucose does. Fructose metabolism occurs in the liver only. In excess, it contributes to triglyceride formation (a type of fat that is a risk factor for heart disease), and a greater risk of fatty liver disease.[8] Excess fructose in the diet from high-fructose corn syrup (HFCS) and fructose-rich fruit juice has also been linked to heart disease, metabolic disease, and obesity.[9,10]

High-Fructose Corn Syrup (HFCS) is a commonly used, highly processed sweetener, which is added to soft drinks and many processed foods. It is a cheap sweetener, hence its high prevalence in American markets. High-fructose corn syrup contains about 55% fructose and 45% glucose. However, don't forget that simple table sugar also contains 50% fructose and 50% glucose. Don't be tricked into thinking that by avoiding high-ructose corn syrup and choosing other sweeteners like cane sugar, even if organic, you are avoiding the health consequences of too much sugar in the diet. Ultimately, all sweeteners will contribute to excess calories and increased risk of weight gain and diabetes. Any sweetener containing fructose consumed in excess can contribute to unhealthy liver effects.

Nature has provided many naturally-occurring sweet foods: vegetables like carrots, bell peppers, sweet potatoes, squashes, and snap peas; spices like cinnamon; and of course, the wide variety of available fruits. There is also the option of choosing small amounts of less processed sweeteners when cooking and purchasing food, instead of the commonly highly processed sweeteners. It is important to consider the amount, quality, and sourcing of the sweetener you choose. Let's visit these options:

Honey is a nutritious sweetener that provides a trace amount of vitamins, minerals, antioxidants, and enzymes. Produced by bees who feed on the nectar from flowers, honey contains both fructose and glucose. Commercial store-bought honey is often heated, pasteurized, and filtered to make the honey look nice and clear in the bottle to the consumer. We recommend raw honey, which hasn't been heated, preserving more of the phytonutrients and enzymes that make honey medicinal. Check your farmers' markets and neighborhood grocers for organic, local, raw honey.

Agave nectar is from the *Agave americana* plant, which grows in South and North America. Agave nectar was initially thought to be a great option for those with blood sugar issues because of its lower level of glucose. However, because it consists of up to 75% fructose, anyone with concerns regarding liver health or triglyceride levels

Don't be tricked into thinking that by avoiding high-fructose corn syrup and choosing other sweeteners like cane sugar, even if organic, you are avoiding the health consequences of too much sugar in the diet.

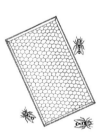

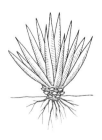

should use agave nectar with caution. In addition, although it does come from a plant and is considered a natural sweetener, agave nectar often undergoes extensive processing. It has been used historically in ceremonies to make tequila.

Maple syrup is the collected sap from sugar maple trees, which is then boiled and reduced to create a rich syrup. It is a combination of glucose and sucrose (a combination of glucose and fructose), making it a relatively low fructose sweetener, with trace amounts of potassium, zinc, magnesium, manganese, calcium, and amino acids. Avoid *table syrup*, which is made of substitute sugars, often high-fructose corn syrup. Notice that real maple syrup costs significantly more than the highly processed table syrup. It may take up to 43 gallons of collected sap to make one gallon of syrup!

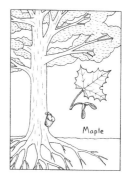

Cane Sugar is from the tall perennial grass native to the Southern tropic regions. It consists of sucrose (a combination of glucose and fructose) and is made from refining the cane plant. Refined white cane sugar is the most common and is heavily processed. Brown sugar is slightly less refined cane sugar without the molasses removed. Examples of even less refined sugar cane is turbinado sugar and evaporated cane juice, which is crystallized sugar cane juice with minimal additional processing. Sucanat and rapadura are the closest variation of raw sugar cane. They have the highest amount of molasses of all of the sugars, which gives them a higher vitamin and mineral content.

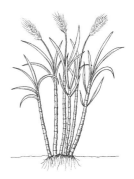

Molasses is removed during the creation of many of the sugars listed above. Molasses can be used as a mild sweetener and provides vitamins and minerals such as iron, calcium, magnesium, and potassium.

Stevia is from the leaves of the native South American plant, *Stevia rebaudiana*, commonly referred to as *sweet leaf*. Calorie-free, stevia does not contain fructose or glucose and therefore does not elicit a reaction in the body like sugar does. It contains a natural chemical called glycoside that creates a strong sweet reaction on the taste buds, but it does not stimulate insulin release. Stevia has been

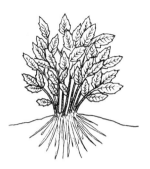

shown to improve insulin resistance by reducing the rise of insulin after eating.[11] Therefore, it can safely be used for people with diabetes and blood glucose regulation problems, although it should not be considered an alternative to medical care for these conditions. It is much sweeter to the taste than sugar, so very little is needed in foods. Be sure to check your label for 100% stevia. Stevia is also being used as a sugar alternative in making calorie-free sodas and beverages without artificial sweeteners.

Sugar Alcohols include erythritol, xylitol, sorbitol, and mannitol. Small amounts of sugar alcohol are found in raw fruits and vegetables and normally pose no health concerns in the natural state. Xylitol contributes very little calories but may be poorly absorbed by the body, causing potential for digestive distress. It has also been shown to be protective against cavities and is commonly used in toothpastes and chewing gum for this reason. Erythritol is also found naturally in some fruits. The body can fully absorb erythritol, causing less potential digestive distress, and it does not contribute calories to a meal. In the diet food industry, erythritol is made by the fermentation of yeast with glucose. The brand name, Truvia®, is a combination of erythritol and Stevia. Erythitol is currently used in many calorie-free beverages, such as Vitamin Water Zero®.

Artificial Sweeteners

In the last few decades, there have been numerous animal research studies observing the relationship of artificial sweeteners and cancer. The results from these studies have not prompted the FDA to recommend reducing or avoiding these sweeteners in the diet. However, many health professionals are convinced that they should not be included in a healthy diet. For instance, daily consumption of diet drinks containing artificial sweeteners has been associated with a 36% greater risk for metabolic syndrome and a 67% increased risk for Type II diabetes.[12] It is ironic that many people are choosing to drink artificial sweeteners thinking it may help to prevent these diseases.

It is important to become familiar with the unusual names of common artificial sweeteners found in our food supply. These artificial sweeteners are used in many energy drinks, diet foods, chewing gums and toothpaste:

Saccharin (Sweet N Low®) has been linked to bladder cancer in lab animals.[13] Saccharin is about 300 times sweeter than sucrose (table sugar), but has a bitter aftertaste. **Acesulfame potassium,** another artificial sweetener that resembles saccharin in structure and taste, is found in many diet foods and chewing gum.

Aspartame (NutraSweet® and Equal®) has been linked to brain cancer, leukemia, and lymphoma in animal studies.[14] Recalling our study of labels in Chapter Five, we learned that aspartame is considered an excitotoxin and can negatively impact neurological functioning in some individuals. Aspartame is forbidden for people with phenylketonuria because of their inability to safely metabolize the chemical.

Sucralose (Splenda®) has been heavily researched, and study results showing negative health effects remain inconsistent. A recent study showed elevated blood sugar and insulin levels following ingestion of Splenda®,[15] which is an interesting find since this is a non-caloric sweetener often chosen to reduce blood sugar and insulin levels. Drinking Splenda-sweetened beverages can actually *increase* one's risk of insulin resistance over time. Splenda is considered an organochlorine. Other well known organochlorines include the not so appetizing chemicals DDT and digoxin, one of the most poisonous substances known to humans. Splenda® is made from sucrose with the addition of chlorine, generating 600 times the sweetness of sugar.

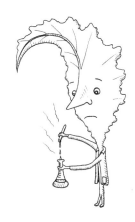

Artificial sweeteners are sometimes hundreds of times sweeter than table sugar. Repeated daily intake of strongly sweet food and drinks can influence long-term desire for very sweet things.

I Need To Lose Some Weight. Shouldn't I Be Drinking Diet Soda Instead Of Real Soda?

Diet sodas are sweetened with the artificial sweeteners listed above. Drinking diet soda may, in the short term, decrease daily caloric intake. However, studies actually suggest an association between drinking diet soda and weight *gain*, as well as the development of Type II diabetes.[16,17,18]

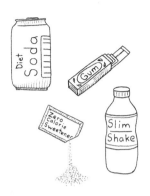

Drinking diet soda may, in the short term, decrease daily caloric intake. However, studies actually suggest an association between drinking diet soda and weight gain, as well as the development of Type II diabetes.

Some people substitute diet soda for regular soda in an effort to reduce caloric intake, but this only adds to a tendency toward further sugar craving and sweet dependence. Artificial sweeteners are sometimes hundreds of times sweeter than table sugar. Repeated daily intake of strongly sweet food and drinks can influence long-term desire for very sweet things.[19] This side effect of influencing one's palate for sweet things may even be transferred from a pregnant woman to her baby, if she is consuming artificially sweetened beverages.[20] *Always remember the healthiest beverage is pure water.*

The FAME series and Dr. Briley weaned me off my diet soda habit. Learning how unhealthy it is for people was very thought-provoking and made me seriously question the value of having it in my home and on the road, enough so to quit the habit.

—Scott, FAME series, Charlee's Kitchen

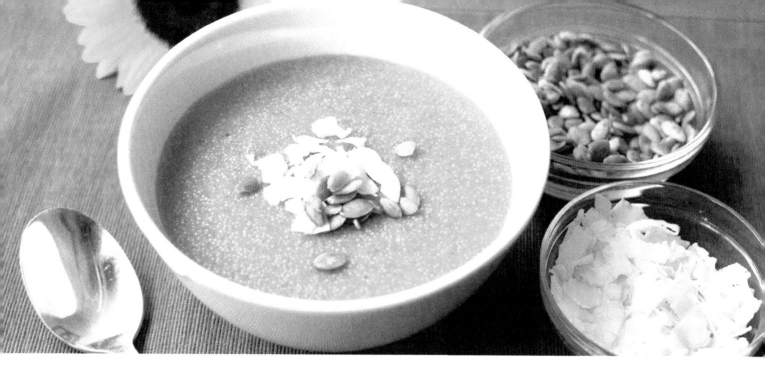

CHAPTER TEN

Benefits Of Breakfast

We started eating oatmeal every morning and cutting out the sugary cereals. My husband started feeling more energized and more refreshed for his long days of work and school. Oatmeal is now his favorite breakfast.

—Christine, ECO project, Mt. Olivet

THE WORD BREAKFAST IS A COMPOUND OF *BREAK* AND *FAST*, DESCRIBING IN ITSELF THE END OF A FAST (ABSTINENCE FROM FOOD or drink) from the night before. Depending upon when dinner was eaten, most people have been fasting for ten to twelve hours prior to breakfast time. If food is not eaten upon awakening, the fast is lengthened, as are the potential negative side effects of prolonged fasting, which can include fatigue, mood changes, and head-aches, including migraines.[1] Eating within one hour of waking is ideal to give the body the fuel it needs to start functioning optimally and to jump-start metabolism.[2] While breaking a fast has numerable noted health benefits, it is equally important to have a fast to break: this means no late night eating or snacking. At least ten to twelve hours nightly with no caloric intake is recommended to reap the benefits of breakfast.

Breakfast provides numerous benefits:

- **Successful maintenance of weight loss**
  Fad diets are initially successful in helping people to shed pounds, but when they stop the diet, weight loss is difficult to maintain. Eating breakfast is a key factor in a successful weight loss maintenance program.[3]

- **Increased focus, decreased stress, better work performance**[4]

- **Improved mood**
  Skipping breakfast can contribute to feelings of fatigue, irritability, or sadness. The body is built to regulate blood sugar levels to the brain, but after a long night of fasting, your brain may not get the fuel it needs to optimally function. Fatigue and irritability may be a sign of low blood sugar. Give the brain some tender loving care and load up on healthy morning fuels—protein, fats, and fiber-rich foods.

- **Increased longevity**
  The Georgia Centenarian Study, which tracked hundreds of older Americans from 1988–2009, studied which lifestyle habits influenced longer than average life span. Regular breakfast eating was a noted habit among this selective group.

- **Decreased risk of heart disease**[5]

- **Decreased risk of developing diabetes**[6]
  Breakfast eaters tend to manifest healthier eating patterns for the remainder of the day, decreasing their risk of developing dangerous blood sugar imbalances over time.

The food with which you choose to break the fast is also important. Aim for a healthy balance of PFFs (protein, fats, and fiber-rich foods) to provide slow fuel. Starting your day with a high dose of sugar and caffeine is a good way to experience a mid-morning crash.

Breakfast And Children

If you have or care for children, there are many reasons to be a good role model and to encourage them to enjoy a healthy meal in the morning. Lack of breakfast or a nutrient-poor breakfast may result in a nutritionally inadequate diet for some children, negatively influencing learning and health in a number of ways.

Consider these reasons for kids to eat a daily breakfast that includes healthy food choices rather than sugar-rich options:

- **Reduced risk of developing obesity**
  Young breakfast eaters have been shown overall to consume more calories in the day compared to non-breakfast eaters. Yet, they maintain a healthier metabolism. This supports the notion that eating breakfast stimulates metabolism for the rest of the day by turning on the *thermic effect of food* (the energy required to absorb, digest, and break down the consumed food).[7,8,9]

- **Improved nutritional intake, including important minerals and vitamins**[10]
  Breakfast provides a strong foundation to grow healthy children into healthy adults.

- **Improved alertness and mood at school**[11]
  Your child's teacher will thank you!

Non-breakfast Eaters—Stay Tuned!

These strategies will help you to incorporate this incredibly healthy behavior into your life.

- Go to bed 15 minutes earlier and wake up 15 minutes earlier in the morning so that there is extra time in the morning to prepare breakfast.

- Make extra dinner the night before or package up left-overs to eat the next morning.

- Plan ahead: make a big batch of oats on Sunday and divide into seven servings for the week and store in the fridge.

- Make twelve hardboiled eggs to *grab-and-go* during the week.

- Remember, eating something is still better than eating nothing. If you have to grab-and-go, consider a handful of nuts and a piece of fruit until you can eat a more complete meal.

Lack of breakfast or a nutrient-poor breakfast may result in a nutritionally inadequate diet for some children, negatively influencing learning and health in a number of ways.

Healthy Breakfast Options

Now, let's list some examples of a healthy, balanced breakfast. Much like fueling an engine, good sense would have us put high quality fuel in our bodies that is guaranteed to provide long-term energy. This type of *slow* fuel will support a healthy metabolism and a more positive mood for the remainder of the day. Remember that *protein, fat, and fiber (or PFF's)* provide slower burning fuel compared to refined carbohydrates. Think of how common it is to see people eating on the go for breakfast with a bagel (refined carbs) or pastry (refined carbs) and a coffee (often flavored with added sugar). It is no wonder that many people feel a mid-morning or mid-afternoon crash in energy due to their poor morning fuel choices.

The following healthy breakfast options include protein, fat, and fiber. If breakfast has always been sweet, then we encourage some experimentation with more savory options.

- **Scrambled eggs** cooked in healthy fats (olive oil, coconut oil, or butter) with your favorite veggies such as spinach, tomatoes, and garlic (see recipe, **Egg and Veggie Scramble**).

- **Unsweetened yogurt** with berries, ground flaxseed, and nuts.

- **Whole-wheat toast** with almond butter and an apple or a pear.

- **Oatmeal** with almond butter or nuts, ground flaxseed, and raisins (see recipe, **Not Just Oatmeal**).

- **Any cooked whole grain** can make a great warm porridge; try quinoa, brown rice, or millet. (See recipe, **Pumpkin Pie Amaranth Porridge**).

- **Apple slices** dipped in nut butter.

- **Bacon** with sautéed vegetables on the side and a piece of fruit.

- **Chia seeds** soaked in almond or coconut milk (at least 30 minutes) with nuts and chopped fruit.

*Remember that **protein, fat, and fiber (or PFF's)** provide slower burning fuel compared to refined carbohydrates. Think of how common it is to see people eating on the go for breakfast with a bagel (refined carbs) or pastry (refined carbs) and a coffee (often flavored with added sugar).*

- **Hard boiled eggs and a piece of fruit.**

- **Dinner for breakfast**! Leftovers! This may include a chicken breast, fish, or beef with steamed veggies or rice and beans with sliced avocado.

- **Smoothies** with frozen berries, dark greens, and nut butter! (See recipe, **Breakfast Smoothie**).

Enjoy breakfast!

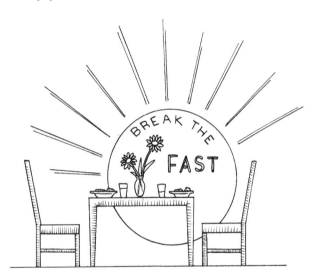

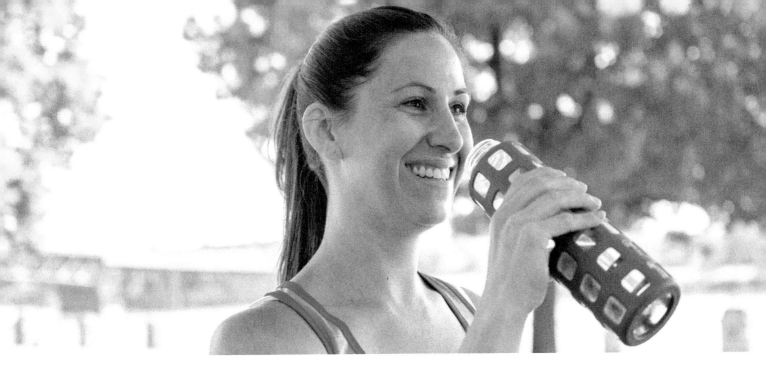

CHAPTER ELEVEN

Habits For Health

A HEALTHY LIFE IS BUILT UPON A COMBINATION OF HEALTHY HABITS. HERE WE EXPLORE SOME ESSENTIAL HEALTHY HABITS THAT will complement healthy food choices. Consider the following aspects of one's lifestyle and how they affect health and well-being: family, friends, intimacy, sense of community, spirituality, recreation, time in nature, fulfilling work or career, service, play, and laughter. All of these are important to cultivate in addition to the Habits For Health we will discuss here: breathing, movement, water, and sleep.

Water

The body is composed of 60% to 70% water. Essential for human life, water helps the body to hydrate, to detoxify, to maintain alertness, to regulate body temperature, and to protect and support joints and organs. Symptoms such as fatigue, mental fogginess, headaches, and dry skin can be improved and often solved with better hydration.

Most adults lose about 1.5 liters of urine daily. An additional liter of water is lost through breathing, sweating, and bowel movements. Food can provide about 20% of total fluid intake, especially watery fruits and vegetables like cucumbers, tomatoes, and watermelon.

While there is no hard and fast rule for how much water a person needs, a simple way to assess if you are well hydrated is to consider the amount and color of your urine. After the first morning's urine, the urine should be clear and copious for the remainder of the day. A more specific recommendation is based on body size: as mentioned earlier, drink half your body weight, measured in pounds, in ounces of water each day. For example, if you weigh 150 pounds, you would aim for 75 ounces of water a day. With exercise, pregnancy, illness, and breastfeeding, more water intake is necessary. Consider drinking eight additional ounces with every 30 minutes of exercise.

All humans need access to clean water. City water systems will make drinking water safe for consumption but often include certain chemicals like chlorine and fluoride. Additionally, very minute amounts of pesticides, herbicides, pharmaceutical medications, and harmful minerals such as lead can make their way into drinking water. **Keep in mind, bottled water will cost extra money and contribute to landfill waste without necessarily making your water safer. Bottled water may or may not have been sourced from the tap.** Additionally, plastic bottles can contribute to the chemical BPA leaching into drinking water. We recommend accessing information about your city's drinking water, which provides background on where the water is sourced and the amount of mineral content, including chlorine and fluoride. Consider a home water filtration unit to help minimize some of the harmful exposures found in drinking water.

Sleep

Sleep is essential to good health. While sleeping, the body recovers from the stress of the day. The immune system becomes active to help fight off infections and to help the body detoxify. Most adults need around 7 to 9 hours of sleep a night, while young children and teenagers may need 10 to 14 hours. *Insomnia* is a form of sleep disturbance lasting at least one month, characterized by difficulty initiating or maintaining sleep, and resulting in clinically significant distress or impairment to normal daytime functioning.

If you weigh 150 pounds, you would aim for 75 ounces of water a day. With exercise, pregnancy, illness, and breastfeeding, more water intake is necessary. Consider drinking eight additional ounces with every 30 minutes of exercise.

Up to 30% of the U.S. population may suffer from insomnia. Women report more sleep abnormalities than men.

People tend to report increased insomnia with advanced age, **although it seems to be related to poor health in older people rather than to the aging process.** Aging is no excuse for poor sleep.

Chronic insomnia is also associated with weight gain.[1] The quality and quantity of sleep will impact the ability to lose and maintain weight loss. Sleep deprivation leads to an increase in a hormone called ghrelin, which increases cravings for sweet carbohydrates. It also leads to an increase in the stress hormone, cortisol, which impacts blood sugar balance, and over time can lead to insulin resistance and weight gain.[2] Until one optimizes this essential habit, it will be difficult to achieve your weight loss goals.

For those struggling to achieve optimal, restorative sleep, note these strategies:

- **Create a routine around sleep and wake cycles** that will help you get the most benefits for your health. Go to sleep at a consistent time every night, optimally before midnight, and wake at the same time every morning.

- **Sleep in a dark room.** Melatonin is a hormone that supports healthy sleep and is activated by the brain during darkness. To promote healthy melatonin production, sleep in a completely dark room (use a sleep mask or black out curtain if needed) and avoid all artificial lights and electronics at least one hour before bed. In addition, expose yourself to bright, natural light for at least 15 to 20 minutes daily.

- **Avoid all caffeine after noon.** Some people may need to avoid all caffeine, while others may need to stop their consumption by 10 a.m, for example. The effects of caffeine can last up to 20 hours for some people. Sources of caffeine include sodas, energy drinks, black or green tea, chocolate, and some over-the-counter drugs.

- **Avoid alcohol.** A glass of wine or a beer may initially aid

Sleep is essential to good health. While sleeping, the body recovers from the stress of the day. The immune system becomes active to help fight off infections and to help the body detoxify. Most adults need around 7 to 9 hours of sleep a night, while young children and teenagers may need 10 to 14 hours.

sleep, but alcohol actually disrupts the brain's ability to enter deeper levels of restorative sleep. In addition, alcohol contributes to unnecessary caloric intake.

- Use the bed for sleeping and intimacy only. A bed is no substitute for the office.

There are a variety of natural medicine tools to support healthy sleep. These tools may include **herbal medicine**, **homeopathy**, **nutritional supplements** (including **amino acid therapies** to promote optimal neurotransmitter function in the brain), and **lifestyle counseling**. Do not wait long to address insomnia. You need and deserve refreshing Z's every night. Your body and brain depend on it.

Breathing

When we consider that breathing is essential to life, it is surprising how little emphasis we place on the quality of breathing and its impact on a healthy lifestyle. Breathing is one way the body detoxifies through the exchange of oxygen and carbon dioxide. Focusing on deep, quality breaths (*diaphragmatic* breathing) can reduce stress and support a healthy blood pressure.[3,4] Deep breathing is really quite simple.

Find a quiet place to sit down or lie down, whichever is most comfortable. Place one hand on the belly. Begin by exhaling all breath through the nose or mouth. Then, take a deep breath in through the nose, for a count of five. Hold the breath for one more second. Exhale for a count of five and wait for one second before beginning the cycle again. Breathe in this rhythm for several minutes. Try to extend your focused breathing practice to ten minutes a day.

During times of stress, simply do a handful of these deep breaths as a reliable stress reduction technique. Deep, mindful breathing before meals and before sleeping can assist optimal digestion and a more restful night of sleep.

Movement

Just like healthy eating, a habit of daily movement is critical for well-

Breathing is one way the body detoxifies through the exchange of oxygen and carbon dioxide. Focusing on deep, quality breaths (diaphragmatic breathing) can reduce stress and support a healthy blood pressure.

A growing body of research shows that long periods of physical inactivity (rather than simply lack of exercise) raise the risk of developing heart disease, diabetes, cancer, and obesity. Those most at risk are sitting eight-plus hours a day, and women are more at risk than men. Each hour spent watching TV is linked to an 18% increase in the risk of dying from cardiovascular disease.

being. In today's fast-paced, technologically-driven world, there are many challenges to incorporate movement into our lives. Many adults sit all day at work. Kids sit all day at school when their physical education classes and recesses are shortened or even cut. With few exceptions, technology (TV, computers, tablets, smart phones) encourages a sedentary lifestyle as well. So, until local and federal educational policy changes and corporate wellness programs for working adults are the norm, it will be up to individuals and families to make sure everyone is physically active.

However, a workout at the gym won't solve it all. It is not just exercise we are promoting; our society is fighting *sitting disease*. The act of sitting for extended periods of time is now recognized as its own risk factor for disease, regardless of the amount of *exercise* in your day. A growing body of research shows that long periods of physical inactivity (rather than simply lack of exercise) raise the risk of developing heart disease, diabetes, cancer, and obesity.[5] Those most at risk are sitting eight or more hours a day, and women are more at risk than men. Each hour spent watching TV is linked to an 18% increase in the risk of dying from cardiovascular disease. Metabolic changes, such as increased triglyceride levels and decreased HDL levels (both of which raise the risk for diabetes and heart disease), as well as decreased carbohydrate metabolism, may occur within one hour of sitting.[6]

What can be done to combat *sitting disease*? It is really quite simple: It is essential to integrate movement into your routine activities. Consider the following suggestions:

- Set a timer to remind you to move your body every 45 to 60 minutes. Stretch, do simple full body exercises to your ability (squats, planks, or yoga, for example), climb the stairs for five minutes, or go for a walk around the building. This is not just at work; do this at home, if sitting on the couch for extended periods, in the car (stop driving first), and even on vacation.

- Stand more instead of sitting! You can read, talk on the phone, answer emails, have meetings, and watch TV, all while standing. Consider a standing desk.

- Walk up the stairs. Avoid elevators.

- Park at the back of the parking lot.

- Carry groceries to your car instead of pushing the cart.

- Bike to work or to run errands instead of driving.

- Enjoy gardening, yard work, and cleaning as forms of daily movement.

- Reduce screen time. Remember, every hour spent in front of the TV, computer, tablet, or smartphone is one hour less of moving. Children who watch TV more than four hours a day have an increased risk of obesity.[7]

- Play with your kids: go biking, play tag, go for a neighborhood walk, play sports, swim. There is no limit.

- Remember, the most basic movement—walking—has many health benefits associated with it, including improved heart and lung function. It is also one of the best ways to reduce fatigue and improve mood.[8] It is an inexpensive activity to do, requiring only time, space, and a pair of comfy shoes. If interested in living a longer, more active life, pick up your gait![9]

Depending on the level of daily activity, most people will still need times of focused exercise in addition to the suggestions listed. Exercise needs to include cardio, stretching, weight-bearing, and strength training. It also needs to include activities that one enjoys to keep motivated. At a minimum, adults should be moving their bodies 60 minutes daily. Kids need one to two hours of movement daily.

Depending upon the level of daily activity, most people will still need times of focused exercise in addition to the suggestions listed above. Exercise needs to include cardio, stretching, weight-bearing, and strength training. It also needs to include activities that one enjoys to keep motivated. At a minimum, adults should be moving their bodies 60 minutes daily. Kids need one to two hours of movement daily. The benefits of movement for kids includes improved mental focus, better performance in school, improved weight and body image, and overall feeling of wellness. Parents are in the best position to serve as healthy, active role models for their children, but so are older siblings and friends. If family members are involved, it can be encouraging for others to participate.

Beyond the physical benefits of moving, there are numerous mental and emotional benefits to incorporating movement into your life including reduced anxiety and depression for all ages.[10,11]

Many of these activities sound basic: drinking water, sleeping, breathing, and moving. Perhaps because they sound so basic, many people do not put much time into thinking how they incorporate these activities into their daily lives. Unfortunately, the consequences of neglecting these activities have come at a great cost to our long-term health. You cannot realize the full benefits of a highly nutritious diet unless other lifestyle habits are in place. For instance, symptoms of dehydration can often appear as hunger pain, making one more likely to grab a sugary snack. Deep breathing helps to tonify the *rest and digest* phase of the nervous system, supporting healthy digestion and allowing for optimal nutrient absorption. Without a restful night of 7 to 9 hours of sleep, it is very difficult to maintain a healthy metabolism and to fight off sugar cravings. Regular movement supports the maintenance of lean muscles, and lean muscle mass is essential for balancing blood sugar over time. These habits for health do require some initial attention and commitment to incorporate into your life, but they are well worth the effort.

Regular movement supports the maintenance of lean muscles, and lean muscle mass is essential for balancing blood sugar over time. These habits for health do require some initial attention and commitment to incorporate into your life, but they are well worth the effort.

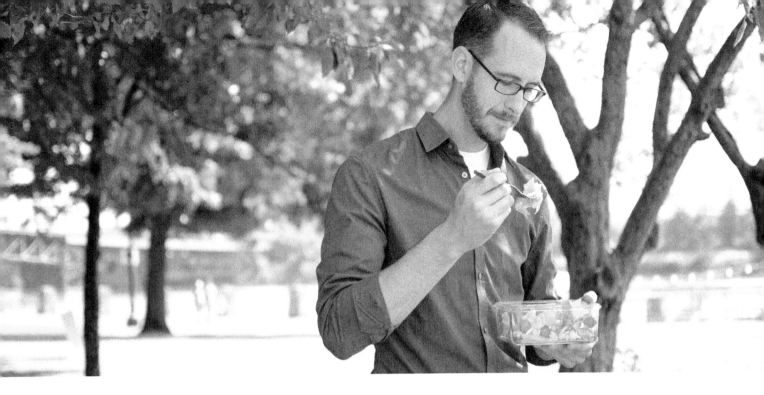

CHAPTER TWELVE

Healthy Eating On The Go

IS IT POSSIBLE TO EAT HEALTHY AT A FAST FOOD RESTAURANT? FAST FOOD TENDS TO BE HIGH IN CALORIES (WITH MORE THAN 50% of those calories coming from saturated and trans fat), and low in nutrients (iron, calcium, riboflavin, and vitamins A and C).[1] Eating just one meal at a fast food restaurant can provide all your daily caloric needs, but little of your daily nutrient needs.[2] Herein lies the problem with fast food: *too many calories, not enough nutrition*.

The consequences of eating fast food go beyond the excess calories. The concept of *fast food* challenges all that we have learned about healthy digestion. It is difficult to remain in a *parasympathetic state* (rest and digest) while eating on the go. In addition, eating fast, fatty foods low in fiber can lead to digestive distress like bloating and gas. Frequent trips to the *fast food nation* also puts one at greater risk for depression, making it that much harder to find the motivation to make healthy lifestyle and dietary changes.[3]

Think about this: as you move along the dietary spectrum from a highly processed diet to a whole foods based diet, how can you visit a fast food restaurant and decrease the negative effects on your health?

Making The Most Of Fast Food

If you are going to find whole foods at a fast food restaurant, salad bars or packaged salads may be the best bet in this department. Look for whole fruits, vegetables, whole grains, eggs, and grilled (not fried) meat at a salad bar or on the menu. You can find a few fast food restaurants that source high quality pasture-raised and hormone-free meat, poultry, and animal products.

Eating a burger without the bun is another way to avoid a highly processed part of a typical fast food meal. In addition to the refined grains and poor quality oils and sugars in a bun, there are added chemicals, preservatives, and artificial flavors. Read the ingredient list below for a bun and beef patty from a popular fast food restaurant to determine the amount of processing:

100% BEEF PATTY— Ingredients:

100% Pure USDA Inspected Beef; No Fillers, No Extenders. Prepared with Grill Seasoning (Salt, Black Pepper).

PREMIUM BUN —Ingredients:

Enriched Flour (Bleached Wheat Flour, Malted Barley Flour, Niacin, Reduced Iron, Thiamin Mononitrate, Riboflavin, Folic Acid), Water, High-fructose Corn Syrup, Yeast, Barley Malt Extract, Soybean Oil, Salt, Wheat Gluten, Contains 2% Or Less: Soybean Oil, Calcium Sulfate, Ammonium Sulfate, Yellow Corn Flour, Conditioners (Sodium Stearoyl Lactylate, DATEM, Ascorbic Acid, Azodicarbonamide, Distilled Monoglycerides, Monocalcium Phosphate, Enzymes, Calcium Peroxide), Turmeric, Annatto and Paprika Extracts (Color), Natural (Plant Source) and Artificial Flavors, Caramel Color, Calcium Propionate (Preservative), Sesame Seed

Contains wheat

Eating a burger without the bun is another way to avoid a highly processed part of a typical fast food meal.

When eating out, limit saturated fats found in fried foods, sausages, or bacon. Fast food restaurants rarely purchase meat made from animals that were raised in their natural environments. Therefore, the quality of the fat in the meat may be less than optimal in terms of its fatty acids profile.

Other ways to make the most of your fast food experience:

- **Seek out whole grains and legumes** to improve the fiber content of your meal. Some fast food restaurants offer brown rice instead of white rice. Fiber-rich legumes in the form of refried beans or black beans may be an option, as well.

- **Drink water with your meal**, not soda. Avoiding all soda (including diet), juice, and sweetened tea is one of the best decisions to make when eating out at fast food restaurants. Consider adding lemon to tap or soda water for taste.

- **Limit mayonnaise, ketchup, creams, and dips**, because these often contain high-fructose corn syrup and unhealthy fats. Remember that salad dressings are often made from omega-6 rich oils, like soy and corn. Mustard can often serve as a healthier condiment.

- **Slow down. Eat with intention.** Pay attention to the environment and how it makes you feel. Take some deep breaths before eating.

- **Avoid supersized and adult-sized portions**, because of the high caloric nature of fast foods. For instance, a twenty-four ounce vanilla milkshake has 600 more calories than a twelve ounce milkshake.

- **Be bold! Ask for the ingredient list and nutrition data.** Take ownership of what food is being ordered.

A Special Note About Saturated Fat

When eating out, limit or avoid saturated fats found in fried foods and highly processed meats like sausages, bacon, and ready-made meat products. Fast food restaurants rarely purchase meat made from animals that were raised in their natural environments. High dietary intake of saturated fat from highly processed meat is linked to heart disease and early death.[4,5] On the other hand, saturated fat from healthy animals and plants can be a part of a healthy diet when combined with other whole foods. However, unless a fast food restaurant is providing information about the ways the animals were raised to produce the meat they sell (and this may include labels like *organic* or *hormone-free* or *free-range*), a fair assumption is that the animals were raised on a soy or corn-based diet in cramped quarters with little exercise.

What About Salt And Sodium?

Remember: Salt is a combination of macrominerals the body depends upon to function. Salt is composed of sodium and chloride. These are important electrolytes in the body that influence regulation of blood pressure, fluid balance, and even nerve conduction. The concern with fast food is excessive amounts of refined salt. Recall that the general recommended daily limit of sodium intake is about 2,300 mg of sodium per day, or *one* teaspoon of table salt, for most people and possibly lower for those at risk of high blood pressure, heart, or kidney disease. Additionally, a diet that contains about twice as much potassium as sodium helps to support healthy heart function. Since the best sources of potassium are fresh fruits and vegetables, eating a fast food diet creates a difficult environment to find a healthy balance of these minerals.

When eating fast food, a good rule is—***do not*** add salt to your food. Don't forget about getting more potassium in your diet to balance out that sodium. Aiming for half a plate of vegetables at each meal will help to provide a balance between sodium and potassium. Here's a shout to the mighty avocado, which contains up to 700 mg of potassium in one medium-size fruit!

Sea salt generally contains the same amount of sodium compared to highly refined table salt. However, sea salt is less processed and does contain other minerals such as calcium, magnesium, and potassium. Do not be misled into thinking you are drastically reducing your sodium intake by switching to sea salt. If you are seeking more flavor, start exploring by adding spices such as cumin, turmeric, oregano, and garlic, for example.

The concern with fast food is excessive amounts of refined salt. . . .Since the best sources of potassium are fresh fruits and vegetables, eating a fast food diet is a difficult environment to find a healthy balance of these minerals.

Final Thoughts On Fast Food

We have been encouraging the development of a healthy relationship with whole, low-processed foods. We are promoting a lifestyle that encourages a slow, steady courtship with **real** food, and we are sure your physical and mental health will improve. If you are a fast food restaurant aficionado, you may have a tough road ahead cultivating this new relationship. Lack of will-power is *not* the reason that many people are unable to stop eating fast foods. It is because fast foods are convenient, readily available, cheap, and contain high amounts of sugar, salt, and fat that are all highly addictive.[6] There are no direct numbers about how often is too often to spend eating fast food. We do know that reducing the frequency of visits to fast food restaurants and eating more fresh-cooked meals at home has been shown to reduce the incidence of obesity.[7] Thus, reducing the frequency of visits is a good start. And by all means, order water not soda.

One of the best ways to reduce your fast food frequency is to be prepared for the day. Don't skip meals—you risk low blood sugar and increased cravings for quick, sugary and salty food. Stay hydrated as dehydration can mimic hunger. Instead of a fast food restaurant, stop at a grocery store and pick up salad and rotisserie chicken, for example. To combat fast food stops due to hunger, prepare for the week ahead on Sundays by creating grab-and-go options by hard-boiling a dozen eggs or by prepping chopped veggies and fruit and packing them in individual containers. To keep your blood sugar stable and your taste buds pleased, create your own fast food opportunities by stocking your car, briefcase or desk with healthy nuts, trail mix, and nut butters.

We do know that reducing the frequency of visits to fast food restaurants and eating more fresh-cooked meals at home has been shown to reduce the incidence of obesity.[7] Thus, reducing the frequency of visits is a good start. And by all means, order water not soda.

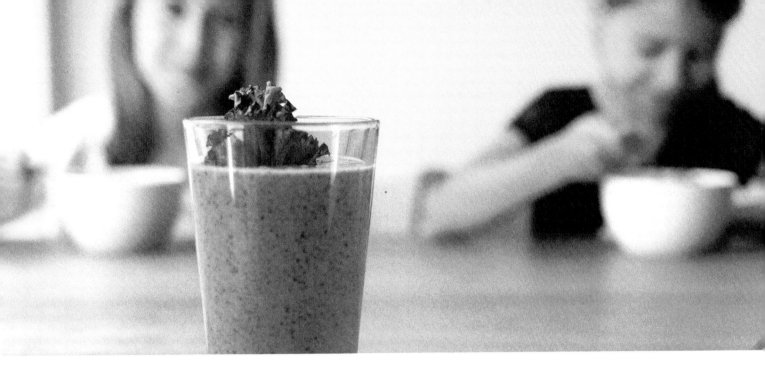

CHAPTER THIRTEEN

Nutritious Lunches And Snacks

It was so interesting to see what my children would try and how they really wanted to go to ECO workshops. Now that they've learned about eating less sugar, I see them making that choice. How to read food labels, learning about fake sugars, choosing which foods are most important if you want to go organic—you can't go over all that too often. It's kind of like gardening. They can tell you what to do, and maybe you'll do it. But when they give you seeds, all you have to do is plant them.

—Ginean (mom), son, age 6, and daughter, age 4, ECO project, Mt. Olivet

I now know more than most people my age about my overall well-being. Now that I have these strategies of being healthy, I can carry it on throughout my whole life. KALE CHIPS ROCK!

—Claire, age 14, FAME series, Charlee's Kitchen

SNACKS CAN BE IMPORTANT FOR BOTH ADULTS AND CHILDREN. THEY HELP BALANCE BLOOD SUGAR AND CAN PROVIDE EXTRA nutrition for the body. Meals and snacks should be balanced in the same way, with protein, fat, and fiber. Most conventional and packaged snacks tend to be high in carbohydrates; for example, crackers, chips, pretzels, and cookies. They also tend to be high in added sugars and can contain trans fats. Snacks that are from whole foods with minimal processing and no additives are better choices.

Some people may not need to snack and can maintain a healthy blood sugar balance by eating three meals a day. For others, five to six smaller meals or a combination of larger meals and smaller snacks may be best. We often think of snacks as being for kids, but adults often benefit from the same healthy snack suggestions.

The key to creating healthy snacks that kids will love is to make them as fun, simple, and engaging as possible. This is true for most adults, too.

Healthy Snacks For Everyone

Fruit and veggie kabobs

Use shish kabob skewers and create a colorful fruit kabob with strawberry, kiwi, pineapple, grape, apple, or pear. Or, make vegetable kabobs out of carrots, zucchini, onion, bell peppers, and mushrooms. Eat them raw with hummus or add olive oil and seasonings and roast them. Kids will love to help make these!

Ants on a log

Take celery sticks and spread nut butters (try peanut, almond, or cashew butter with no sugar added) and line raisins across the top.

Frozen fruits

Frozen fruit is available year-round, or buy fresh fruits in season and freeze them yourself. Try frozen grapes or a bowl of frozen berries for dessert, or add them to unsweetened yogurt. (See recipe, **Coconut Berry Bliss**.)

Smoothies

Freeze ripe bananas without the peel. Use them in smoothies with frozen berries and milk (try coconut, almond, or hemp milk). Blend them for an ice-cream like treat. You can add nut butter for an excellent protein breakfast and ground flaxseeds to add fiber. (See recipe, **Breakfast Smoothie**.)

"My 17-year old son and I are taking the ECO project classes for a school health credit. I have learned so much, even if the info is not brand new, it comes at a time when I am making a more focused effort regarding our diet at home. We have definitely increased our intake of vegetables and whole grains. Experimenting with whole grains has been fun. The actual cooking part of the class makes trying new things so do-able. I think this is such an effective way to teach and actually affect changes in everyday life."

—Jody, ECO Project, Mt Olivet

Carrots, sugar snap peas, celery, red peppers, and cucumber can be dipped in hummus or other dips and offer a fun activity for kids.

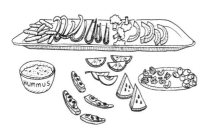

Spiced nuts

Almonds, walnuts, cashews, and filberts (hazelnuts) are all great choices. Enjoy them raw, or roast them yourself.

Veggies

Fresh vegetables should always be on hand for quick snacks. Take 15 minutes to chop all of your vegetables so they are ready to grab-and-go. There are pre-chopped, pre-washed, bagged veggies available if time is an issue, although they will be more expensive to purchase. Carrots, sugar snap peas, celery, red peppers, and cucumber can be dipped in hummus or other dips and offer a fun activity for kids.

Veggie dips

Choose dips without trans fats or high-fructose corn syrup. Hummus and guacamole are great options. Carrots and celery taste great dipped in nut butters.

Trail mix

Make your own by mixing your favorite nuts, seeds, and dried fruits with no sugar added. The bulk section of the grocery store is a great place to find a variety of ingredients and to purchase the amount needed. Check the labels on pre-made trail mixes to avoid added sugar.

Turkey roll-ups

Spread hummus on a slice of deli turkey. Add a thin slice of cheese or avocado and a few pieces of spinach or lettuce and roll it up. These are easy to pack in lunches or to enjoy as a good protein snack. (See recipe, **Turkey Roll-up.**)

Freeze-dried fruits and veggies

These are great for a crunchy snack. There are freeze-dried strawberries, blueberries, mangoes, sweet peas, tomatoes, bananas, and plantains that can be found at almost all grocery stores. Make sure there are no added sugars or preservatives.

Granola bars

Read the ingredients. Look for fiber content, sources of added sugar, and trans fat. The healthy options are usually made of whole nuts, seeds, whole grains, and dried fruits (See recipe, **Coco Loco Protein Bars**.) Stay away from *high protein bars* which have highly processed sources of protein (whey and soy) and are far from a whole food. These bars are not a substitute for meals.

Any snacks with refined sugar should be kept for special occasions rather than daily indulgences.

Healthy Lunches

Along with breakfast, lunch is the meal that provides kids and adults the energy needed to focus and learn in school or at work. Lunch contributes to balanced blood sugar later in the day, reducing evening cravings.

A balanced lunch will include whole grains or starchy vegetables, protein and healthy fat (meat, nut butter, beans), and at least one to two servings each of fruit and vegetables.

For kids and adults used to having something sweet in their daily lunch, try shifting to packing their favorite fruit. Avoid packing juice, candy, or foods with high amounts of sugar or any high-fructose corn syrup. For kids, getting a special note from a loved one can be a fun and healthy alternative.

Lunch Ideas To Get You Started

Nut Butter and Banana Jam Sandwich (PB and J)

You are never too old for a good ol' PB and J. Try this alternative to sugar-sweetened jelly (See recipe, **Nut Butter and Banana Jam Sandwich**.) Spread mashed bananas (banana jam) and nut butter (peanut, almond, or cashew with no-sugar added) on 100% whole grain bread. Sunflower seed butter is a great alternative that is high in vitamin E. You can also substitute a local, raw honey in place of banana jam.

Any snacks with refined sugar should be kept for special occasions rather than daily indulgences. High-fructose corn syrup should be avoided at all times, if possible. Limit or avoid fruit juices, because they are a concentrated form of natural sugars (and some manufacturers add more pro-cessed sugar).

(Honey should not be given to infants under 12 months of age.) If you use a premade jam or jelly, look for one with no added sugar or high-fructose corn syrup.

Hummus Hero

Hummus is rich in protein, fat, and fiber and comes in a variety of consistencies and flavors (plain, spinach, garlic, red pepper, sun-dried tomato, etc.). Make your own! (See recipe, **Homemade Hummus**.) Hummus is a great dip for fresh veggies or in place of mayonnaise on a 100% whole grain sandwich.

Lox Lunch

Layer lox (fillet of brined salmon) or smoked salmon, spinach, cream cheese, and tomato on a slice of whole-grain bread, or a bagel, and enjoy.

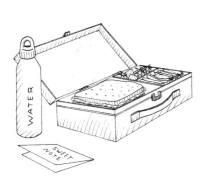

Sandwich Wrap

Add turkey, chicken, fish, beef, or tempeh with your favorite vegetables (spinach, lettuce, cucumber, avocado) and roll them in a whole grain tortilla or a blanched green leafy vegetable, such as collard greens.

Egg Salad

Mix hard boiled eggs with mayonnaise (without trans fat) and mustard and serve over a bed of greens with veggies. Or, pack separately to spread on whole grain crackers or as a dip for sliced carrots and celery.

Brown rice and beans

Season to taste with salt and cumin. Serve alone or in a whole grain tortilla with chopped tomato, lettuce or spinach, and avocado.

Dinner leftovers

Any recipe for a dinner can make for a healthy lunch option. Prepare extra and pack into lunch containers.

Some Fun And Tasty Ways To Prepare Veggies

Root vegetable fries

Yams, sweet potatoes, carrots, and parsnips can be cut into fry shapes. Place them in a baking dish and mix with avocado oil or melted coconut oil or butter. Spice with salt, pepper, rosemary, or oregano. For a sweeter option, spice with cinnamon or nutmeg. Bake at 350°F for 30-45 minutes until soft. Kids love baked root veggies! (See recipe **Baked Root Fries**.)

Steamed Carrots

Steam baby carrots or cut carrots until soft. Add butter, coconut oil, or olive oil and serve.

Cheesy Trees

Steam broccoli until soft and sprinkle a small amount of grated cheese on top. Or, use another healthy fat (olive oil, coconut oil, butter) and a little salt. Makes a great side dish.

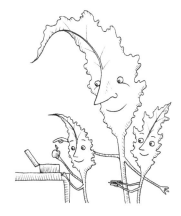

Getting Kids On Board With Healthy Eating

If there are children in your life, teaching them how to eat and enjoy healthy foods is just as important as teaching them to ride a bike, swim, read, and climb a tree. Food provides them with nutrients to support their body in order to accomplish physical and mental activity. But, that doesn't mean that choosing healthy foods comes naturally to children, especially when there are so many options and heavy exposure to kid-centric marketing of junk food. The time it takes to encourage, model, and empower kids to eat healthy foods is worth the effort. Caregivers have the power to exert great influence on their little one's eating habits.[1,2,3] Take the role seriously, and find like-minded support with other health-focused adult eaters. Be inspired by the fact that modeling healthy eating habits with little ones will influence the health of future generations. Let children be a part of the process by helping with making the grocery list, going shopping, and preparing the meal.

Set the expectation clearly with children that healthy eating is important, and be consistent with this message. This does not mean one has to be a rigid, rule maker and enforcer of consequences for poor eating choices. Rather consistent adult role modeling of healthy eating behaviors is priceless. It will be an easier road to travel if there is support in the home to make healthy eating a lifestyle.

People tend to use food as a reward for accomplishing a task, whether it be completing a project, getting a good grade, or scoring a goal at soccer, for example. This strategy introduces the concept of emotional eating by enforcing the idea that it is okay to eat unhealthy foods when doing something good. People may also use food for comfort when they experience many other emotions: anger, sadness, loneliness, boredom, and feeling anxious or stressed.

Set the expectation clearly with children that healthy eating is important, and be consistent with this message. This does not mean one has to be a rigid, rule maker and enforcer of consequences for poor eating choices. Rather, consistent adult role modeling of healthy eating behaviors is priceless. It will be an easier road to travel if there is support in the home to make healthy eating a lifestyle. But, if you find yourself the lone wolf of healthy eating in your home, stay the course. Your commitment can reduce the risk of childhood obesity and other related diseases, and that is a worthwhile effort.[4]

Some Ideas To Get You Started

Give options

Allowing kids to choose between two food options, either for a snack or something to pack in their lunch, is empowering. However, if giving a child an option of a bowl of ice cream or a salad, don't be surprised when the majority of children choose the ice cream. Our taste buds prefer foods with sugar, salt, and fat.

Give the child a choice, but offer two healthy options. It can become overwhelming if a child has too many options, so keep it to two or three at the most.

Avoid using food as a reward or as a bribe

If a *sweet treat* (ice cream, cookies, cake) is used as a reward for finishing another healthy food—broccoli, for example—the child will increasingly prefer the *sweet treat* and learn to dislike the healthy food.[5,6] In addition, this strategy gives the impression that there is something undesirable about broccoli. People also tend to use food as a reward for accomplishing a task, whether it be completing a project, getting a good grade, or scoring a goal at soccer, for example. This behavior introduces the concept of *emotional eating* by enforcing the idea that it is okay to eat unhealthy foods when doing something *good*. People may also use food for comfort when they experience many other emotions: anger, sadness, loneliness, boredom, and feeling anxious or stressed. These patterns are sometimes learned from a very young age and reinforced in our culture as people mature. In these cases, it is important to address the underlying emotions in order to be successful at making changes in dietary patterns.

It is important to understand that not all emotional connections to food are negative. Many cultures and traditions revolve around this concept of celebrating with food (birthday cakes, holiday sweets, candy and chocolate giving for Valentine's Day). While it isn't necessary to cut out all celebrations and rewards, be aware of the frequency of their occurrence. As a culture, we can begin to shift the focus toward creating traditions, celebrations, and communities that come together with an emphasis on healthy food.

If an occasional sweet treat is desired, don't allow it to be dependent on finishing another food item. Remember that fresh or frozen fruit or smoothies can be a great *sweet treat* and still a healthy choice. In addition, a special treat or reward doesn't have to be a food item.

Similar to using food as a reward, we often see families bribing the child to eat certain foods by promising something in return. If a child is told that he can watch TV, or stay up later after eating a certain food item, the transaction makes the healthy food seem undesirable and a chore to eat. Bribery will *not* encourage healthy food behaviors.[7]

The best course of action is to model healthy eating for children to observe.

Avoid hiding junk food

Some parents think that it is a good idea to hide the *junk food* so that a child won't eat it. Many homes have a hidden stash of candy in a locked drawer or placed high upon a shelf. Unfortunately, most kids pick up on this strategy. If the childen know that a certain food is being hidden from them, it will increase their desire to eat that food even more, as it may seem more special, exciting, forbidden, or something just for adults.[8]

Store all your food the same way, and be open with children about which foods in the cabinet are healthy food choices and which foods should only be eaten on occasion.

Some parents think that it is a good idea to hide the junk food so that a child won't eat it. Many homes have a hidden stash of candy in a locked drawer or placed high upon a shelf. Unfortunately, most kids pick up on this strategy. If the child knows that a certain food is being hidden from them, it will increase their desire to eat that food even more, as it may seem more special, exciting, forbidden, or something just for adults.

Limit hiding or masking healthy food

If hiding or dousing healthy food with something else (large amounts of ketchup or ranch dip, for example), or hiding puréed vegetables in other dishes, kids will not learn to like the taste or texture of that food.[9]

While dips can be a fun and healthy way for kids to try new foods such as vegetables, consider the quality of the dip and the amount; aim to serve appropriate portion sizes. If you are *hiding* vegetables in other dishes, (e.g. pureed spinach in tomato sauce) consider giving a serving of that vegetable on their plate, too, so they can be visually and texturally introduced to that food.

Introducing Foods

A child is more likely to eat a food if it is introduced multiple times. It is not uncommon for a child to refuse to even try certain foods at first. This is completely normal and does not indicate a special child who simply doesn't eat vegetables.[10] Parents and caregivers: hang in there and continue to offer healthy foods to these young eaters. With older children, explain that the goal is to try new foods, not that they have to like each new food. A healthy food such as kale or carrots may need to be introduced up to *ten times* before a child becomes familiar and comfortable including the new food in his/her diet.[11] Persistence and commitment to providing healthy foods for children will have long term positive benefits on their health. If there is one thing to remember about trying to feed a child: do not force him/her to eat. Share words of inspiration and motivation and work to commit to this important food journey with your young ones.

Don't use bribery or rewards when introducing new foods; just continue to be a good role model and accept that they may refuse the food at first. Also, texture, flavor, and presentation are important when introducing foods. Some kids will eat plain steamed broccoli but not want broccoli in a stir-fry with sauce on it. Experiment with cooking and seasoning in different ways and know that it may take time, patience, and an adult enjoying a big plate of broccoli with a smile.

Don't use bribery or rewards when introducing new foods; just continue to be a good role model and accept that they may refuse the food at first. Also, texture, flavor, and presentation are important when introducing foods. Experiment with cooking and seasoning in different ways and know that it may take time, patience, and an adult enjoying a big plate of broccoli with a smile.

Use Positive Reinforcement

Parents will give positive reinforcement to kids for learning how to get dressed, tying their shoe, sharing toys, and during potty training. It is just as important (and often overlooked) to give positive acknowledgement when children choose and eat healthy foods. Children today are bombarded with food choices and extreme marketing of junk food. Making healthy choices can be challenging for kids (let's be honest, it can be hard for adults, too). So, let us congratulate each other when we eat our vegetables or try a new food.

Give high fives! Tell them how strong and healthy they will be by eating their nutritious meal. Let a child overhear you telling someone else how well they ate their healthy dinner. This will boost their confidence and empower them to continue to make healthy choices.

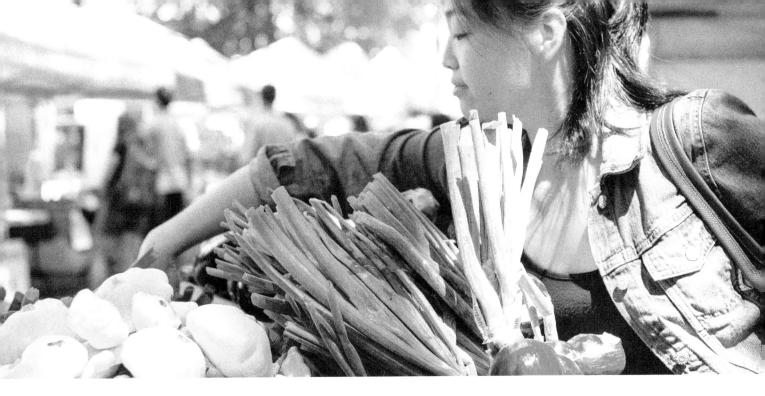

CHAPTER FOURTEEN

Shopping Guide And Everyday Superfoods

I look at food differently, now. I have gratitude for the farmers and stores that take a risk to produce organic, whole foods. I cook differently now with new spices, and lots of them, and better-for-me oils. Bread is NOT a staple anymore. Oatmeal as granola was phenomenal as were the smoothies—what a surprise! Lastly, I look at NDs differently—with greater love and reverence because of your compassion, knowledge, and creativity.

—Susan, FAME series, Charlee's Kitchen

IT IS TIME TO CONVERT WHAT WE HAVE LEARNED INTO ACTION. LET'S HEAD TO THE GROCERY STORE! THIS CHAPTER FOCUSES ON how to navigate a conventional grocery store. Conventional grocery stores remind us just how highly processed our food supply can be. This chapter will highlight strategies to use at the grocery store to make the healthiest and most economical purchases. As you move toward a whole foods lifestyle, you may need to begin with small steps.

General Grocery Shopping Tips

Read these tips before you head out to shop:

- Do not go shopping while hungry; buying on impulse and purchasing unhealthy foods or larger portions is more likely.

- Always make a list before going to the grocery store. List the meals to be made and the staple foods needed. You will be less likely to overspend and make impulse purchases. Making a list will help prevent returning to the grocery store for a forgotten item.

- Allow for flexibility when buying produce, taking into account what is in season or on sale.

- At the store, start by purchasing food at the periphery—that is often where the most nutritious foods are, such as fruits and vegetables, fresh meat, poultry and fish. Then go to the aisles or bulk section where you can locate whole grains, legumes, and nuts. Limit shopping in the aisles where there are pre-packaged or pre-prepared foods.

- When products that the family uses often are on sale, buy extra. Bulk grains and beans last for many months in your pantry and refrigerator, as long as they are stored properly. Do not buy extra sale items if you are not likely to use them often.

- Be aware of the placement of less healthy food products that promote impulse buying for you or your children.

- When comparing the ingredient list between different brands, also include a price comparison by checking the price per unit, often shown as the price per ounce.

How to shop the bulk section

One of the benefits of shopping in bulk is that it allows experimentation of new foods and spices at minimal risk to the pocket book. Shopping in bulk can help you stick to a budget. Buy exactly the amount you need for a specific recipe instead of buying double that amount in pre-packaged items. Proper containers to store your bulk foods will

> "
> *The FAME series helped me shop better—I'm not afraid of the bulk section anymore. And who knew I could make my own almond butter, all natural, no added ingredients, to use instead of peanut butter?*
> —Shannon, FAME series, Mt. Olivet

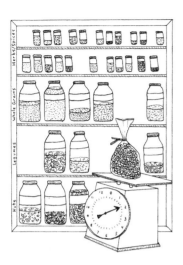

be needed. Clean and reuse bottles or containers (preferably glass ones). Rinse them out, take off the label, and fill them with bulk items. This will prevent food from spilling out of the bags and will keep them free of pests. Designate an area in your pantry and fridge for specific bulk food items.

Common bulk items to purchase

- *Dry beans* can be up to three times cheaper than canned beans. In addition, preparing beans at home eliminates added salt, sugar, or preservatives found in canned beans.

- *Whole grain* prices can vary. It's usually beneficial to compare the packaged prices to the bulk prices. Keep in mind that bulk grains allow you to purchase specific amounts. Whole grains can be stored in a cool dark place, like a fridge or freezer.

- *Flour* is also available in the bulk section and is often less expensive than packaged flour. Always look for whole grain flour. Be sure to have a storage plan for the flour at home; the thin bulk bags at most stores will not allow for proper storage of bulk flour. In particular, store all flour in air tight containers in a cool, dark place; either the fridge or freezer. Since flour is ground whole grains, there is more potential for spoilage when exposed to light and heat.

- *Herbs and spices* can be purchased in small amounts. This is much cheaper than paying for the entire jar of spices, and bulk purchasing makes trying lots of different flavors easier. If you buy a spice in the jar the first time, save the jar and refill it from the bulk section. Store spices for up to six months, at most, and then refresh.

- *Dried fruits* are often less expensive in the bulk section. Avoid any dried fruits that have added sugar or *sulfites*. Sulfites are a preservative that can have negative side effects ranging from hives to aggravation of asthma in some individuals.[1,2,3,4,5]

- *Raw nuts* may also be less expensive when purchased from the bulk section. It is a convenient way to purchase as much or as little as needed. You can also soak and roast nuts at home. Make your own trail mix by purchasing nuts, seeds, and dried fruit and mixing them at home.

Top Five Everyday Super Food Groups For Your Cart

Most people hear the word *superfood* and think of exotic tropical berries like gogi, acai, or noni berries. While these berries do pack a punch in terms of antioxidants and can be a great addition to the diet, locally grown whole foods from your region are truly daily superfoods. Daily superfoods to keep you healthy:

1. *Vegetables of all types. Top choices for your basket.*

   - *Dark green leafy vegetables (DGL):* Include DGLs as part of your daily diet. They provide minerals, vitamins, antioxidants, and fiber. Dark green veggies are one of the most nutrient-dense foods. Eat both raw and lightly steamed or sautéed greens. Top greens choices include spinach, collards, chard, kale, mustard, and dandelion leaves.

   - *Squash:* Look for the orange-fleshed varieties, which pack more beta-carotene, a vitamin A precursor, than almost any other vegetable or fruit. Gain all the nutritional benefits by adding some healthy fat to the squash. Try mashed squash with butter or coconut oil, cinnamon, and nutmeg.

   - *Cruciferous vegetables:* Cabbage, Brussels sprouts, broccoli, Bok choy, turnips, cauliflower, kale, and collard greens are all members of this family of vegetables. They all contain a healthy dose of phytonutrients, vitamins, minerals, and fiber. They contain sulfur compounds that can help prevent cancer, decrease inflammation in the body, and reduce oxidative stress.[6] The best cooking method for these veggies is steaming or sautéing. Enjoy one to two cups prepared at least three times weekly.

     Cruciferous vegetables have been well-studied for their role in cancer prevention. Female breast cancer survivors who had the highest intake of cruciferous vegetables within

> *We are making better choices when purchasing items at the store. Planning for meals is becoming easier with knowing the correct balance of fats, carbs, and protein.*
>
> —Anne, FAME Series, Charlee's Kitchen

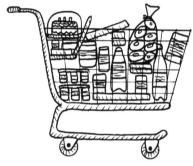

unhealthy cart

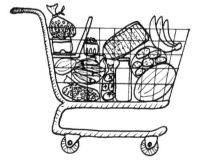

healthy cart

Cruciferous vegetables have been studied for their role in cancer prevention. Female breast cancer survivors who had the highest intake of cruciferous vegetables within the first three years following their diagnosis showed a 62% decreased risk of death associated with breast cancer as well as a 32% decreased risk of cancer recurrence. The more cruciferous vegetables eaten, the lower risk of stomach, lung, colon, and rectal cancer.

the first three years following their diagnosis showed a 62% decreased risk of death associated with breast cancer as well as a 32% decreased risk of cancer recurrence.[7] The more cruciferous vegetables eaten, the lower the risk of stomach, lung, colon, and rectal cancer.[8]

- *Beets:* With their rich, deep color, this root vegetable provides valuable antioxidants and is traditionally known for supporting liver health. Beets are also packed with minerals. As an added bonus, buy beets with the greens attached. Beet greens are edible and are good steamed by themselves or substituted for other dark green leafy veggies in a recipe.

- *Garlic and onions:* These members of the allium family aid in balancing blood sugar, keeping a strong immune system, supporting healthy blood pressure, and supporting detoxification pathways in the body.[9,10] They also make your food taste great.

2. Fruits

Fruits are packed with vitamins, fiber, and antioxidants that aren't found anywhere else in our diet. Remember, fruit juice does not count as a substitute for a whole fruit. Top fruits for the basket:

- *Berries:* Try frozen, fresh, or dried (with no sugar added); any type is great. Berries are thought to provide some of our most potent antioxidants.

- *Citrus fruits:* Lemons, oranges, and grapefruit are high in immune-stimulating vitamin C, as well as antioxidants that are good for vision and liver health. If you are taking prescription medications, ask your doctor if grapefruit consumption is okay for you; grapefruit juice can affect the metabolism of some medications.

- *Melons:* Each variety of melon has a different balance of vitamins and minerals, as well as antioxidants. Cantaloupes, in particular, provide a great amount of vitamin C and beta-carotene.

- *Apples or pears:* Take advantage of the many varieties of apples and pears. Each variety has a different flavor and a different complement of health-boosting antioxidants. Apples have been found to aid in blood sugar balance and cholesterol balance due to their soluble fiber content.[11]

3. Healthy Fats

- *Avocados* contain a rich source of monounsaturated fat, potassium, and fiber.

- *Butter from pasture-raised cows* will be richer in omega-3 fatty acids, vitamin E, and beta-carotene than its conventionally made counterpart.[12,13] Butter can be used to stir-fry and sauté at higher heats and is great for baking.

- *Coconut oil* provides a stable fat to cook with at high heat **and** it contains medium-chain fatty acids, which support a healthy digestive tract and increase metabolism.[14] Coconut oil can easily be substituted for butter.

- *Nuts and seeds:* Choose pecans, almonds, walnuts, and macadamia. Nuts and seeds provide a nutrient-dense package of protein, fat, and fiber.

- *Wild Alaskan salmon*: Salmon provides health-promoting essential omega-3 fatty acids that help to reduce inflammation and promote a healthy brain. It is also a great source of complete protein.

4. Beans and Legumes

Beans are packed with heart-healthy fiber, protein, and vitamins. The more colorful the bean, the higher the antioxidant value.

- Top beans for the basket: black beans, kidney beans, black-eyed peas, and lentils.

5. Fermented Foods

These foods provide the body with healthy bacteria (probiotics) to

Fermented foods provide the body with healthy bacteria (probiotics) to keep the immune system strong and aid in digestion and bowel health.

keep the immune system strong and aid in digestion and bowel health.

- Top fermented foods for the basket: unsweetened yogurt, kefir (a cultured milk beverage), miso, kimchi, kombucha, tempeh, and properly prepared pickles and sauerkraut (not all store-bought sauerkraut is lacto-fermented; most are just in vinegar).

A Final Review Of Foods To Limit Or Avoid

1. Limit excess added and artificial sweeteners

- High-fructose corn syrup (HFCS) is difficult for the liver to process and causes a large spike in blood sugar. Common sources are soda, juices, baked goods, candy, ketchup, and other condiments.

- Aim to avoid all soda and juices, even if they are *natural*, because they provide little nutritional value to the body, only sugar and calories.

- Artificial sweeteners are chemicals created in a lab and are not part of a whole foods diet.

2. Limit refined carbohydrates

This ingredient sneaks up in most packaged foods.

- Refined carbohydrates include sugar and whole grains processed to remove the bran and germ—the most nutritious parts.

- If a package says *enriched* wheat flour or white flour, white rice, sugar, fruit juice, or corn syrup, then the product contains refined carbohydrates.

- These simple sugars provide quick and large spikes in blood sugar. Eating these foods frequently can contribute to the development of obesity and diabetes.

Refined carbohydrates are often grains processed to remove the bran and germ— the most nutritious parts.

- Common sources are *white* foods: store bought bread or buns (unless packaging states 100% whole grain), pre-made baked goods, pasta, white rice, frozen meals, potato chips, and white flour.

3. *Avoid trans fats and partially hydrogenated fats*

    Read all labels for this ingredient.

    - These are oils that have been chemically changed to keep them from becoming rancid.

    - There is no safe amount of trans fat intake.

    - Remember that trans fats do not have to be added to the Nutrition Facts label if there is less than .5 grams per serving. Be sure to read the Ingredient list. If the label shows *partially hydrogenated oils*, then the food contains some level of trans fats.

    - Common sources: packaged snacks (cookies, crackers, and chips), frozen French fries, frozen entrees, margarine and shortening, fast foods, and fried foods.

4. *Limit omega-6 fatty acids*

    - Americans tend to over-consume omega-6 fats from corn, soybean, safflower, and sunflower oils, which are found in packaged and fast foods. These omega-6 fats, while essential to the diet, need to stay in a healthy balance with omega-3 fatty acids, which most people are under consuming.

    - Remember that our sources for omega-3 fatty acids are fish, flaxseed, chia seed, walnuts, and pasture-raised meat and eggs.

5. *Limit highly processed foods*

    - This includes packaged foods such as canned soups, frozen dinners, boxed foods, chips, candy, and pre-made sauces, gravies, and salad dressing.

Remember that trans fats do not have to be added to the Nutrition Facts label if there is less than .5 grams per serving. Be sure to read the Ingredients list. If the label shows partially hydrogenated oils in the list, then the food contains some level of trans fat.

- Highly processed foods may contain high amounts of sodium, sugars, trans fats, preservatives, and artificial colors, flavors and sweeteners, which are hard for the body to process and eliminate.

Stocking The Pantry

The following list can help you build your pantry and fridge with foods that are commonly used at home and in the majority of our recipes. Always be conscious of what produce is in season. Our recipes are generally very adaptable to substitutions.

Please see each individual recipe for a complete list of ingredients.

Top Five Medicinal Spices

Turmeric
Traditionally used in Ayurvedic cooking in combination with black pepper for better absorption; high in curcumin (natural anti-inflammatory), powerful antioxidant, immune stimulant

Cinnamon
High in minerals (iron, calcium, manganese), balances blood sugar, anti-inflammatory, natural sweetener

Ginger
Relieves digestive complaints (nausea, motion sickness, vomiting), immune stimulant, natural anti-inflammatory, pain relief

Cayenne
High in capsaicin, topical and internal anti-inflammatory, blood mover, reduces platelet aggregation, clears congestion

Thyme
High in volatile oils, immune stimulant, anti-microbial, cough suppressant, expectorant, anti-spasmodic

Herbs and Spices
- Black pepper
- Cayenne pepper
- Chili powder
- Cinnamon
- Cumin
- Garlic powder
- Ginger (fresh and/or dried)
- Oregano
- Rosemary
- Sea salt
- Turmeric
- Thyme

Oils and Fats
- Avocado and avocado oil
- Butter
- Coconut oil
- Extra virgin olive oil
- Sesame oil

Whole Grains
- Amaranth
- Brown rice
- Brown rice flour
- Cornmeal
- Millet
- Oats
- Quinoa

Legumes and Peas
- Black beans
- Black-eyed peas
- Garbanzo beans
- Kidney beans
- Green peas
- Lentils
- Pinto beans

Vegetables
- Asparagus
- Bell peppers
- Bok choy
- Broccoli
- Brussels sprouts
- Carrots
- Cauliflower
- Cucumber
- Dark Greens:
    - Chard
    - Collards
    - Dandelion greens
    - Kale
    - Mustard greens
    - Spinach
- Garlic
- Mushrooms (fungus)
- Onions
- Romaine lettuce
- Squash
- Sweet potato
- Tomato (fruit)

Fruits
- Apples
- Bananas
- Berries
- Citrus:
    - lemon
    - lime
    - grapefruit
- Melons
- Pears

Nuts and Seeds
- Almonds and almond butter
- Cashews
- Chia seeds

Nuts and Seeds (cont'd)
- Flaxseed
- Hazelnuts (filberts)
- Peanuts and peanut butter
- Pecans
- Sesame seeds
- Sunflower seeds
- Walnuts

Dairy and Dairy Alternatives
- Almond milk
- Cheese
- Coconut milk
- Unsweetened yogurt

Meat/Fish/Poultry
- Chicken
- Beef
- Fish:
    - salmon
    - cod
    - halibut
- Pork
- Turkey
- Eggs

Other
- Honey
- Maple syrup
- Molasses
- Mustard
- Shredded coconut
- Raisins
- Tamari
- Vinegar:
    - apple cider
    - balsamic
    - rice

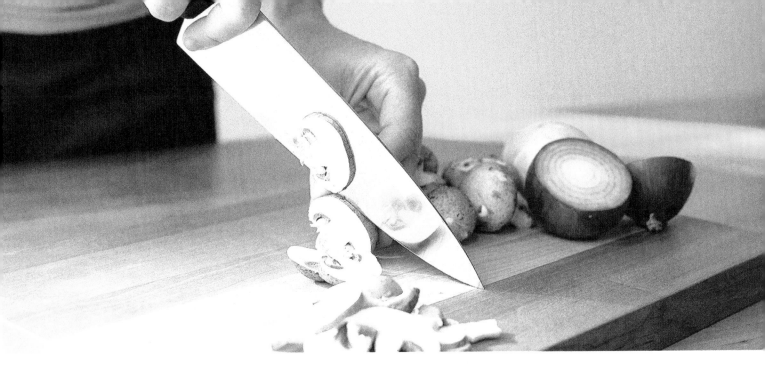

CHAPTER FIFTEEN

Kitchen Skills

The FAME series has helped me bridge the gap between wanting to make more whole-foods meals and actually doing it. The fact that my whole family (3 of us) took the class together was really helpful because we encourage each other at home.

—Elizabeth, FAME Series, Charlee's Kitchen

Instructions For Cooking Whole Grains, Beans, and Greens

Soaking whole grains

To create an acidic environment that begins the breakdown of nutrient inhibitors such as phytic acid, whole grains can be soaked overnight in water with two tablespoons of apple cider vinegar, lemon juice, or plain yogurt. This process makes the grains more digestible and increases the nutrient availability of the grain. Before cooking the grains, simply drain the water, rinse the grain in a colander, and continue with the instructions listed below. Most grains were traditionally prepared this way.

Rinse: Prior to cooking, rinse whole grains thoroughly in cold water until the water runs clear. Then strain to remove any dirt or debris. A fine mesh colander may be needed.

Cook: Boil the water, add the grain, return water to a boil, reduce heat, then cover and simmer until tender.

For ground whole grains (using meal, grits, or flakes):

Combine cold water and grain. Bring to a boil, stirring constantly. Reduce temperature to low, cover and cook to desired thickness.

Test: Check the cooked grain before removing from heat to ensure it is thoroughly cooked. Whole grains should be slightly chewy when cooked.

Fluff: Remove from the heat and gently fluff them with a fork. Cover and set aside for 5 to 10 minutes and then serve.

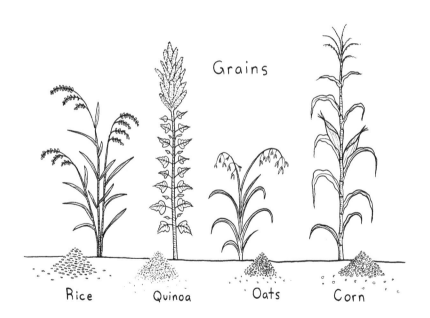

Grains

Rice   Quinoa   Oats   Corn

To create an acidic environment that begins the breakdown of nutrient inhibitors such as phytic acid, whole grains can be soaked overnight in water with two tablespoons of apple cider vinegar, lemon juice, or plain yogurt. This process makes the grains more digestible and increases the nutrient availability of the grain.

Table 15.1 Cooking Guidelines for Common Whole Grains

Grain (1 cup dry)	Cups Water	Estimated Cook Time	Yield (in cups)
Amaranth	2½	20-25 min	2½
Barley, hulled	3	75 min	3½
Buckwheat groats	2	15 min	2½
Cornmeal, coarse ground	4	20 min	2½
Millet, hulled	3	20 min	3½
Oats, rolled	2	15 min	2
Oats, steel cut	3	20 min	3
Quinoa	2	20 min	2 or 3
Rice, brown	2	35-40 min	3
Rice, wild	4	50-60 min	4
Sorghum	3	50-60 min	2½
Teff	4	15 min	3
Wheat, berries	3	50 min	2

Cooking Dried Beans

Rinse: Rinse thoroughly in cold until water runs clear.

Soak: Soaking beans before cooking helps to reduce some of the indigestible compounds (saponins) that can cause gas, and it breaks down phytic acid.

Regular soak: Put beans into a large bowl and cover with 2 to 3 inches of cool, clean water. Add 2 tablespoons of apple cider vinegar, lemon juice, or plain yogurt and set aside for at least 8 hours or overnight; then drain and rinse.

Quick soak: Put beans into a large pot and cover with 2 to 3 inches of cool, clean water. Bring to a boil then boil briskly for 2 to 3 minutes. Cover and set aside, off of the heat, for 1 to 2 hours. Then drain and rinse.

Cook: Put soaked beans into a large pot and cover with two inches of water. Don't add salt at this point since that slows the beans' softening. Slowly bring to a boil, skimming off any foam on the surface (many impurities rise to the top in the foam). Reduce heat, cover, and simmer. Stir occasionally and add more liquid if necessary, until beans are tender when mashed or pierced with a fork. Cooking times vary with the variety, age, and size of beans; generally one to two hours. Refrigerate cooked beans in a covered container for up to four days. Alternately, store them in an airtight container and freeze them for up to six months.

Peas and lentils

Split peas and lentils do not need to be pre-soaked or sprouted, they require less preparation, and are great for meals when you are busy. However, whole dried peas should be soaked overnight.

Rinse: Rinse dried peas and lentils as you would dry beans (see above).

Cook: Bring water to a boil, add the lentils or peas, return to a boil, and then reduce the heat and simmer, partially covered, until tender, 30 to 45 minutes. Some lentils will cook in as little as 15 to 20 minutes.

Cooking tip: Uncooked dried peas and lentils can be added directly to soups and stews, too. Just be sure there is enough liquid in the pot.

See Table 15.2 for information about individual cook times and water requirements. This table is for pre-soaked beans. Beans with an asterisk do not require soaking.

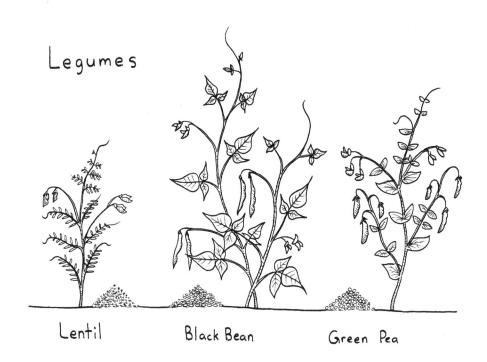

Legumes

Lentil   Black Bean   Green Pea

Table 15.2 Cooking Guidelines for Common Beans

Bean (1 cup dry)	Cups Water	Estimated Cook Time	Yield (cups)
Black beans	4	60–90 min	2¼
Black-eyed peas	3	60 min	2
Cannellini	3	45 min	2½
Fava beans	3	40–50 min	2
Garbanzo (Chick peas)	4	60–90 min	2
Great northern beans	3½	90 min	2⅔
Green split peas*	4	45 min	2
Yellow split peas*	4	60–90 min	2
Kidney beans	3	60 min	2¼
Lentils, brown*	2¼	20–30 min	2¼
Lentils, red*	3	15–20 min	2 to 2½
Lima beans	4	60 min	2 to 3
Navy beans	3	45–60 min	2⅔
Pinto beans	3	60–90 min	2⅔

*Do not require soaking.

Preparing greens

In selecting greens, look for crisp leaves with a bright green color. If the leaves are yellowing, this is often a sign of aging. The greens may contain fewer nutrients and not last as long after purchasing. They may also have an unpleasant taste. Check with your grocer or a local farmer's market to learn the best season to purchase certain greens that are harvested locally in your area. In many parts of the country, the growing season for kale and spinach can extend through winter months, while dandelion leaves may appear in many markets only in the spring. Most greens can be stored in the refrigerator for several days—or better yet, in the crisper drawer of your refrigerator. If you find yourself struggling with the purchasing and storing of fresh greens, consider initially purchasing frozen greens to incorporate into meals. Frozen greens can provide a nutrient-dense boost to smoothies, soups, and stews. We encourage you to explore tasting these different greens in a variety of ways to develop a long-term relationship with these superfoods. See Table 15.3 for preparation tips for common greens.

Cooking With Oils, A Recap

Many of the recipes included in this book recommend using coconut oil, butter, or avocado oil for higher heat needs, such as baking and sautéing. Unrefined coconut oil, butter, and good quality animal fats (lard, tallow) are low-processed saturated fats that have a higher smoke point and a delicious flavor. Unrefined avocado oil is high in monounsaturated fats and has a very high smoke point. In general, any of these fats and oils can be easily substituted for each other in recipes.

Extra virgin olive oil is best used for salad and meal dressings or for low temperature cooking due to its lower smoke point.

Remember to take into account the type of fat (saturated versus unsaturated), the degree of processing, and the smoke point when choosing fats and oils. Saturated fats in general oxidize more slowly due their chemical structure. Polyunsaturated fats are less stable with heat exposure, due to their double bonds. Choose unrefined oils, as they have not been highly processed with heat and chemicals, and they retain more nutrients and flavor than refined oils. Smoke points can vary based on the type and quality of the oil and the processing. They are sometimes listed on the label of the oil. You can also cook many foods at a lower temperature, which will slow the rate of oxidation of the oil.

Limit or avoid refined (highly processed) oils, especially those that are high in omega-6 polyunsaturated fats. Avoid all partially hydrogenated fats and oils.

Use Tables 15.4 and 15.5 as guides to help you choose healthy fats to include in your meals.

Table 15.3 Cooking Guidelines for Dark Green Leafy Vegetables

Variety	What To Expect	Preparation Tips
Arugula	Strong peppery flavor Soft tender leaves	Enjoy raw in salad
Beet greens	Mild flavor, both sweet and bitter Tender leaves	Sauté, stir-fry, or finely chop and add to soups and stews
Bok choy	Sweet, mild flavor Firmer, juicy leaves	Sauté, stir-fry, or finely chop and add to soups and stews
Collards	Mild flavor Tough, thick leaves when raw that soften when cooked	Sauté, stir-fry, or finely chop and add to soups and stews Blanch and use as a wrap for vegetables or stir-fry; cut away thickest part of stem for wraps
Dandelion greens	Small leaves- sweet and mild Larger leaves- tend toward bitter	Enjoy small leaves raw in salad Sauté, stir-fry, or finely chop and add to soups and stews
Kale (Dinosaur/Italian/Lacinato, Green, Purple)	Mild flavor Dinosaur/Italian/Lacinato kale—elongated leaves with a curly edge Green kale—softer, very curly Purple kale- softer, delicate leaves	Choose Dinosaur or Italian kale for kale chip For all varieties: Sauté, stir-fry, or finely chop and add to soups and stews Finely chop and enjoy in salads Add to smoothies
Mustard greens	Subtle spicy mustard flavor, bitter	Steam, stir-fry or sauté, and add to soups.
Spinach	Sweet, mild flavor Soft leaves	Enjoy raw in salad Sauté, stir-fry, or finely chop and add to soups and stews Add to smoothies
Swiss chard (Red, Green, Rainbow)	Sweet flavor	Sauté, stir-fry, or finely chop and add to soups and stews

Table 15.4 Saturated Fats and Their Smoke Points

Fat Or Oil	Things To Know	Type Of Fat	Smoke Point °F
Butter	Organic, pasture-raised/pasture butter is best.	Saturated	350°F
Clarified butter or ghee	Higher smoke point than butter. Commonly used in Ayurvedic cooking. Low in lactose and milk protein.	Saturated	375–485°F (depending on purity)
Coconut oil	Extra virgin/virgin oil (unrefined) is less processed and has a distinct coconut flavor. Refined oil has a neutral flavor. Can also be used for skin and hair care.	Saturated	Extra virgin/virgin (unrefined): 350°F Refined: 400°F
Lard	Rendered fat from a pig. Lard from pasture-raised pigs is the best source.	Saturated	370°F
Palm oil	Increased demand has caused negative environmental impacts. Certified sustainable (CSPO) sources are available.	Saturated	Unrefined: 300°F Refined: 450°F
Tallow	Rendered fat from beef, sheep, deer, and poultry. Tallow from pasture-raised animals is the best source.	Saturated	Beef tallow: 400°F

Table 15.5 Unsaturated Fats and Their Smoke Points

Fat Or Oil	Things To Know	Type Of Fat	Smoke Point °F
Almond oil	Can also be used for skin care.	Monounsaturated	Unrefined: 420°F Refined: 495°F
Avocado oil	Unrefined oil has high smoke point. Can also be used for skin care.	Monounsaturated	Unrefined: 450°F Refined: 520°F
Canola (rape-seed) oil	Highly processed. Common genetically modified organism.	Monounsaturated	400°F
Corn oil	Highly processed. High in omega-6 fatty acids. Common genetically modified organism. Often called *vegetable oil*.	Polyunsaturated	450°F
Cottonseed oil	Highly processed and often partially hydrogenated (trans fat). Used in conventional *vegetable shortening*.	Polyunsaturated	420°F
Grapeseed oil	Highly processed. High in omega-6 fatty acids. Can be by-product of wine making.	Polyunsaturated	392°F
Olive oil	Extra Virgin has low smoke point. Good for dressings.	Monounsaturated	Extra virgin: 325°F Virgin: 400°F
Peanut oil	Unrefined has distinct peanut flavor.	Monounsaturated	Unrefined: 320°F Refined: 450°F
Safflower oil	Highly processed. High in omega-6 fatty acids.	Polyunsaturated	450°F
Sesame oil	Unrefined has distinct sesame flavor.	Monounsaturated	Unrefined: 350°F Refined: 445°F
Soybean oil	Highly processed. High in omega-6 fatty acids. Common genetically modified organism. Often called *vegetable oil*.	Polyunsaturated	450°F

Table 15.5 Unsaturated Fats for Cooking and Their Smoke Points (cont'd)

Fat Or Oil	Things To Know	Type Of Fat	Smoke Point °F
Sunflower oil	Higher in omega-6 fatty acids.	Polyunsaturated	450°F
Walnut oil	Unrefined oil has mild walnut flavor.	Monounsaturated	Unrefined: 320°F Refined: 400°F

RECIPES

All Seasons

Spring and Summer

Fall and Winter

I have been encouraged to pay more attention to, and become more aware of, what I eat and its effect on my body. I've learned that a beautiful, delicious, and nutritious meal can be made from simple, easy to find whole ingredients, and it can be done quickly.

— Sally, FAME Series, Charlee's Kitchen

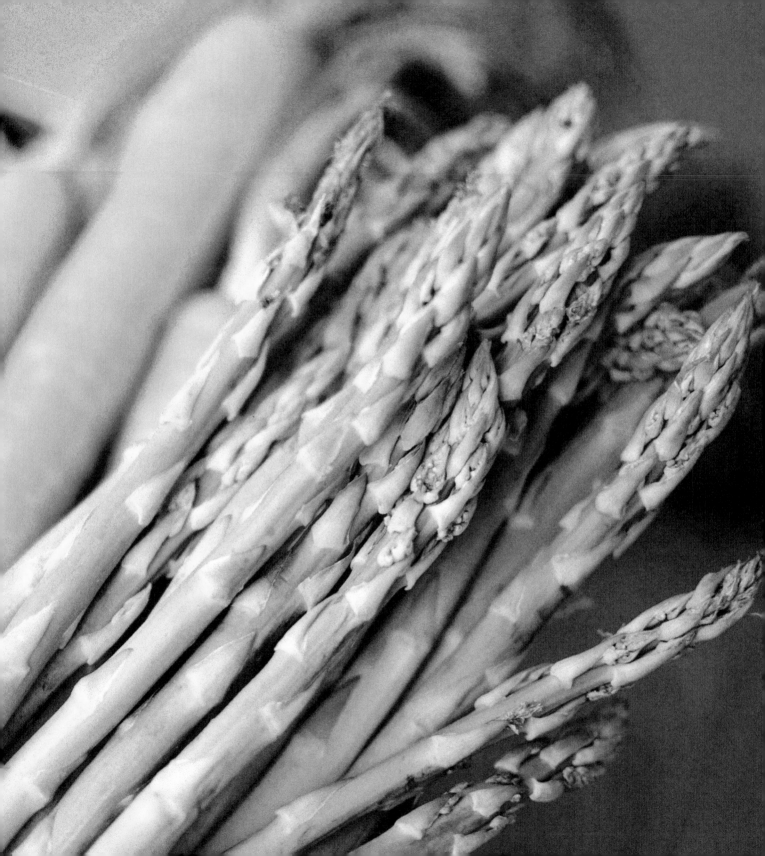

ALL SEASONS

ingredients

1½ cups brown rice

3 cups water for rice

3 cups cooked or canned pinto beans

2 tablespoons coconut oil, lard, or butter

½ yellow onion, diced

4 cloves garlic, peeled and minced

1 tablespoon cumin

½ to 1 teaspoon salt

¼ teaspoon black pepper

1 cup water or low-sodium vegetable broth

2 medium avocados, diced

2 medium tomatoes, diced

¼ cup chopped cilantro

¼ teaspoon cayenne (optional)

1 finely chopped fresh jalapeno (optional)

Servings: 4 to 6

Refried Pinto Beans and Rice

Perfecting brown rice and beans provides you and your family with a wholesome and adaptable meal option that is rich in plant-based protein as well as fiber. The addition of diced tomatoes, avocados, and cilantro provide vibrant color, antioxidants, and healthy fat. Add crunchy kale chips to complete your nutritious plate.

Directions for rice:

1. Add rice and water to a saucepan and bring to a boil.

2. Cover, reduce heat to a gentle simmer, and cook about 35 to 40 minutes until the rice is tender. Do not lift the lid frequently or stir the rice while rice is cooking.

3. Fluff with a fork before serving.

Directions for refried beans:

1. If using dried beans, refer to soaking and cooking methods in Chapter Fifteen, **Kitchen Skills**. If using canned beans, drain and rinse.

2. Heat large saucepan over medium heat and add 2 tablespoons of oil.

3. Sauté onions until translucent, then add garlic and finely chopped jalapeno (optional). Add salt, black pepper, cumin, and cayenne (optional).

4. Add beans and ½ cup water or broth. Allow to heat thoroughly. Then, mash beans well with a potato masher or fork. Add additional water or broth as needed for desired consistency.

5. Serve beans over rice and top with diced avocado, chopped tomato, and cilantro.

Nutrition Facts:

- One serving size is ½ cup cooked beans. Consuming ½ cup of pinto beans a day has been shown to lower levels of total cholesterol and LDL and to improve heart health.[1] Half a cup of pinto beans also provides 7 grams of fiber.

- Combining beans with a whole grain like brown rice provides a complete protein.

- One serving size of whole grain cooked rice is ½ cup. Whole grain rice is rich in fiber, B-vitamins, and trace minerals such as manganese and selenium. Manganese superoxide dismutase, which protects cells from injury, is the primary antioxidant in our cells. Eating one cup of brown rice provides our daily needs of manganese. B-vitamins provide great nutritional support for the nervous system and help to balance mood.

Baked Kale Chips

ingredients

Kale chips are a delicious introduction to this amazing dark green leafy vegetable and can be substituted for potato chips. We find that Italian/lacinato kale works best for these chips, though you can experiment with other varieties.

¾ pound kale (one bunch)
2 to 3 tablespoons melted coconut oil
2 cloves garlic, peeled and minced
½ teaspoon salt
Cayenne pepper (optional)

Directions:

1. Preheat oven to 350°F.

2. Peel kale leaves away from thick stems and cut or tear leaves into equal "chip-size" pieces (approximately three inch by three inch).

3. Mix kale pieces, 2 cloves of chopped garlic, salt and 2 to 3 tablespoons of oil into a bowl and massage together with hands. Spread kale chips evenly in one layer onto baking sheets.

4. Bake for 12 to 15 minutes. Ovens may vary in their baking time. Move kale around on the baking sheet every 3 to 4 minutes to prevent burning and sticking. Bake until kale is slightly crisp around the edges.

Tips:

- Experiment with various spices for your kale chips. Try adding rosemary, oregano, curry powder or nutritional yeast.

Breakfast Smoothie

i n g r e d i e n t s

1 cup frozen strawberries

1 cup frozen blueberries

1 fresh or frozen peeled banana

2 cups unsweetened coconut milk or almond milk

¼ cup ground flaxseed or chia seed

¼ cup sliced almonds or almond butter

2 ounces spinach (1 to 2 large handfuls)

Servings: 4 (1 cup serving)

Smoothies can be a great way to add greens to your morning meal. Nut butters provide an earthy, grounding flavor to this berry-rich meal. Smoothies allow for morning variety while ensuring a delicious opportunity to get whole fruits, green leaves, nuts and seeds into your day. Smoothies can also make a great snack. Be creative. There is no exact science to making a smoothie.

Directions:

1. Place all ingredients into a blender. Blend at high speed until smooth. Add more liquid (water or milk) for a thinner smoothie.

2. Pour in glasses and enjoy.

Tips:

*   Try the following substitutions: Milk (unsweetened hemp milk, rice milk or cow milk); Berries (blackberries or raspberries); Greens (chard or kale); Nuts (use other raw nuts if you have a strong blender), or nut butters (cashew, walnut, or sunflower seed butter).

*   Substitute fruits: apples or pears with ginger and cinnamon for a fall smoothie.

*   Keep in mind that protein powder is generally a highly processed supplement. While it can be a good option for some to add extra protein to your smoothie on occasion, be sure to check the ingredient list on the label and avoid artificial colors, flavors, sweeteners, or other chemical additives. Look for protein powders that contain only one or two ingredients that you can understand clearly, such as brown rice, pea, or hemp protein. Eating whole food sources of protein is always preferred.

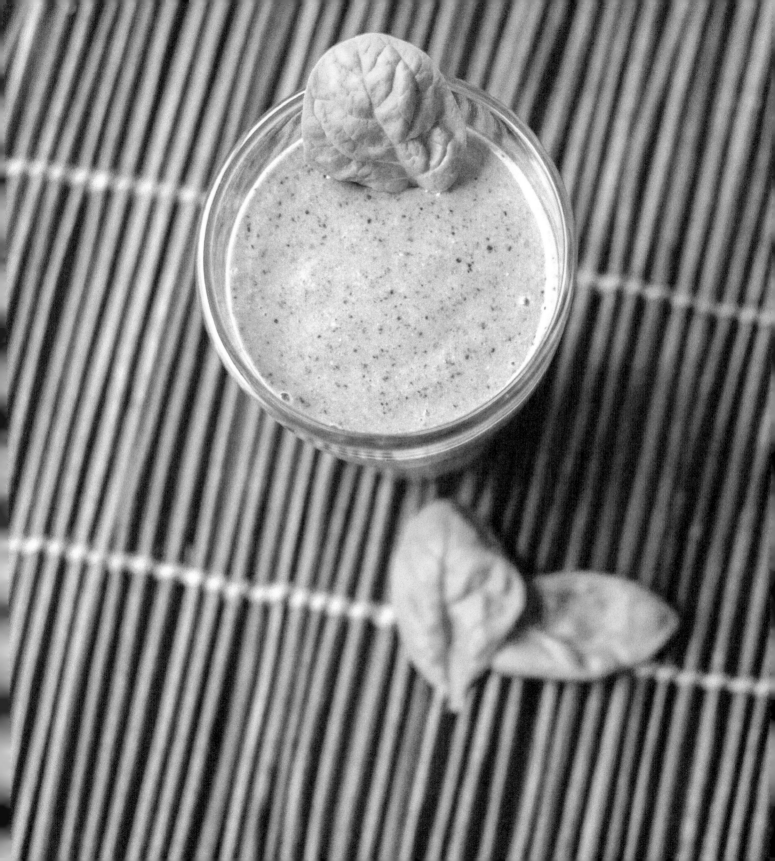

ingredients

Not Just Oatmeal (Rolled Oats)

2 cups rolled oats

4 cups water or unsweetened milk (almond, coconut, dairy)

¼ teaspoon salt

½ cup chopped nuts or 4 table- spoons almond butter

¼ cup raisins

4 teaspoons raw honey

½ teaspoon cinnamon

1 cup blueberries

¼ cup ground flaxseed

Servings: 4

Whole oats are a great source of soluble fiber and have been shown to support healthy cholesterol levels.[2] To increase the amount of healthy fat and protein in your bowl of oatmeal, consider adding ground flaxseed, nuts or nut butters to balance this whole grain meal. Natural sweeteners like honey or fresh fruit can be enjoyed with oatmeal. Both rolled oats and steel cut oats offer similar nutrition to start your day. If you substitute steel cut oats for this recipe, use 1 cup of steel cut oats to 3 cups of water and cook for 15 to 20 minutes.

Directions:

1. Bring water or milk and salt to a boil.

2. Add oats and simmer over low heat for approximately 10 minutes, depending upon desired consistency. Stir occasionally.

3. Take the pot off the heat and let cool.

4. Serve cooked oats with healthy toppings: chopped nuts or almond butter, honey, cinnamon, blueberries, and ground flaxseeds.

Tips:

• One serving size of oats is 1 cup cooked oats.

• Cooked steel cut oats store well in the fridge for up to five days.

• Divide your cooked oats into single portions and have a healthy breakfast ready to go for the rest of your week. Add nuts and flaxseed before eating.

Healthy Chicken Bites

Are you looking for a delicious and fun way to bring a healthier version of chicken *nuggets* and French fries into your home? The following three recipes are perfect ways to get the whole family involved in creating simple and wholesome alternatives to popular fast food items. Chicken is an excellent source of lean protein and B-vitamins for balanced energy throughout the day. Choose chicken that is organic and pasture-raised.

Directions:

1. Preheat oven to 400°F.

2. Melt coconut oil over low heat. Grease bottom of 9" x 13" baking dish with 2 tablespoons of coconut oil. Set aside remaining coconut oil.

3. Cut chicken into *nugget-sized* pieces, and set aside.

4. Add milk and egg to a bowl and whisk together.

5. Place cornmeal and flour with mixed herbs and salt in another bowl and mix together.

6. Dunk chicken pieces first into liquid mixture and then dredge through corn meal and flour mixture until well coated. Place chicken evenly into baking dish and lightly drizzle remaining melted coconut oil on top of battered chicken bites. Place dish into preheated oven and bake for 10 minutes. Flip the chicken bites and bake for additional 10 minutes.

7. After 20 minutes, check to see if fully cooked by cutting a piece in half. If there is any pink meat showing, return to oven for additional time.

4 tablespoons coconut oil

1½ pounds chicken breasts (3 to 4 ounces per person)

¾ cup milk (unsweetened almond, coconut, or dairy)

1 egg

¾ cup brown rice flour

¼ cup fine or medium ground corn meal

2 tablespoons mixed, dried herbs (rosemary, garlic, thyme, oregano)

1 teaspoon salt

Servings: 6

ingredients

Colorful Cole Slaw

*8 to 10 cups finely chopped or
shredded green or red cabbage
(1 small or ½ medium head)*
½ cucumber, diced
1 carrot, diced or shredded
3 asparagus, finely sliced
4 green onions, finely sliced

COLE SLAW DRESSING:
½ cup extra virgin olive oil
2 tablespoons apple cider vinegar
2 tablespoons fresh lime juice
1 tablespoon raw honey
¼ cup finely chopped cilantro
1 to 2 cloves garlic, minced
¼ teaspoon salt
¼ teaspoon black pepper

Servings: 6 to 8

Cabbage can initially be a tough sell for many, but we are sure you will enjoy every bite of this zesty and colorful salad. Make a balanced FAME plate with the **Healthy Chicken Bites** and **Baked Root Fries**.

Directions:

1. In a large serving bowl, combine finely chopped or shredded cabbage, cucumber, carrots, asparagus, and green onions.

2. For the dressing, add all ingredients into a blender. Blend until smooth.

3. Add dressing to cabbage salad so that it is lightly coated and mixes well. Save any excess dressing. Allow salad to marinate for at least 60 minutes before serving.

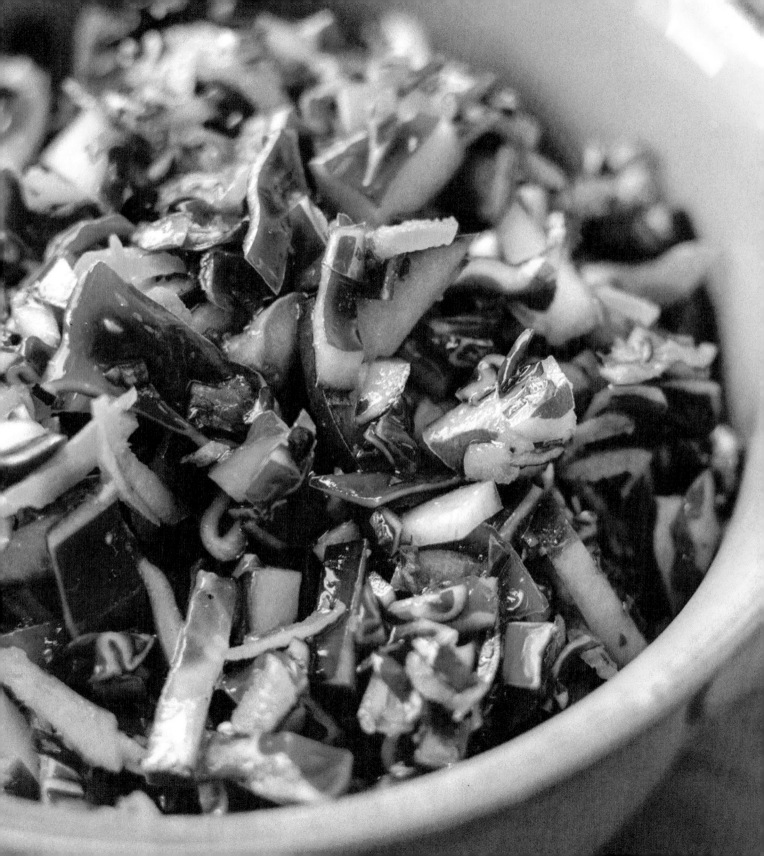

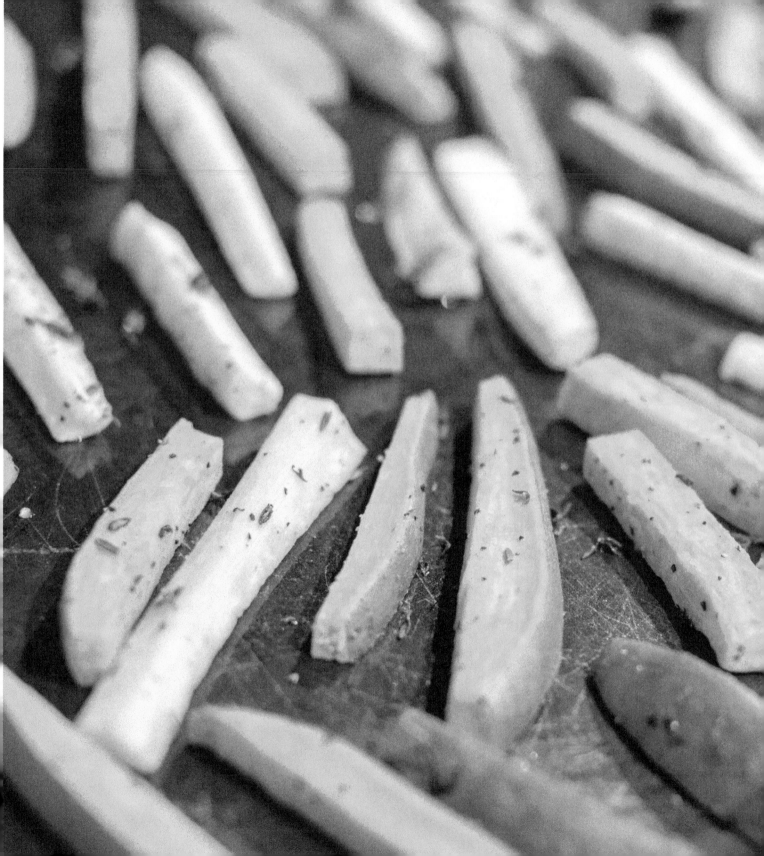

Baked Root Fries

When baking fries, think beyond the white potato. Add more colors and variety with other tasty root veggies and bring a power-packed nutritional punch to this favorite finger food.

Directions:

1. Preheat oven to 400°F.

2. Slice potatoes, carrots, and parsnips into thin wedges or "fries" and place in a bowl.

3. Massage root vegetables with oil. Add salt, pepper, and other spices of choice.

4. Spread evenly on a baking sheet and bake for 30 to 45 minutes. Be sure to stir roots every 15 minutes. Remove from oven when slightly brown and crispy.

Tips:

• Experiment with adding different combinations of spices to your baked root fries; combine cumin, garlic and cayenne, or rosemary and garlic powder. For sweet and spicy flavors, combine cinnamon and cayenne.

i n g r e d i e n t s

2 medium sweet potatoes

2 large carrots

2 medium parsnips

¼ cup melted refined coconut oil or avocado oil

1 teaspoon salt

½ teaspoon black pepper

Cayenne pepper, cinnamon, cumin, rosemary, garlic powder (optional)

Servings: 6 to 8

Baked Salmon Cakes

These sweet and savory cakes are a delicious way to enjoy salmon throughout the year. They provide a rich source of healthy protein and fat and pair well with a basic green salad. When time is limited for meal prep, they are quick to prepare and very satisfying.

ingredients

¾ cup mashed sweet potato

14-16 ounces canned wild salmon

1 egg

¹/₃ cup medium-grind cornmeal or almond meal

3 tablespoons finely chopped fresh parsley

2 tablespoons finely chopped yellow onion

¾ teaspoon paprika

½ teaspoon cumin

½ to 1 teaspoon salt

½ to 1 teaspoon black pepper

4 tablespoons coconut oil

Servings: 4 patties

Directions:

1. Steam sweet potato until soft. Mash well.

2. Remove excess water from canned salmon and add to a bowl. Separate salmon with a fork.

3. Mix together cornmeal or almond meal, parsley, onion, paprika, cumin, salt, and pepper. Add salmon and mashed sweet potato and mix together. Whisk egg in a small bowl and gently combine with all ingredients. Shape into four patties.

4. Heat frying pan over medium heat and add oil. Cook patties for about 8 minutes on each side until lightly browned.

Nutrition Facts:

- Canned salmon will often contain small, delicate and edible bones that provide an excellent source of calcium. We recommend keeping these mineral-rich additions in your recipe. Salmon skin may also be present, which can be a source of omega-3 fatty acids. Be sure to purchase wild-caught salmon to reduce exposure to environmental toxins, which can accumulate in the flesh of the fish.

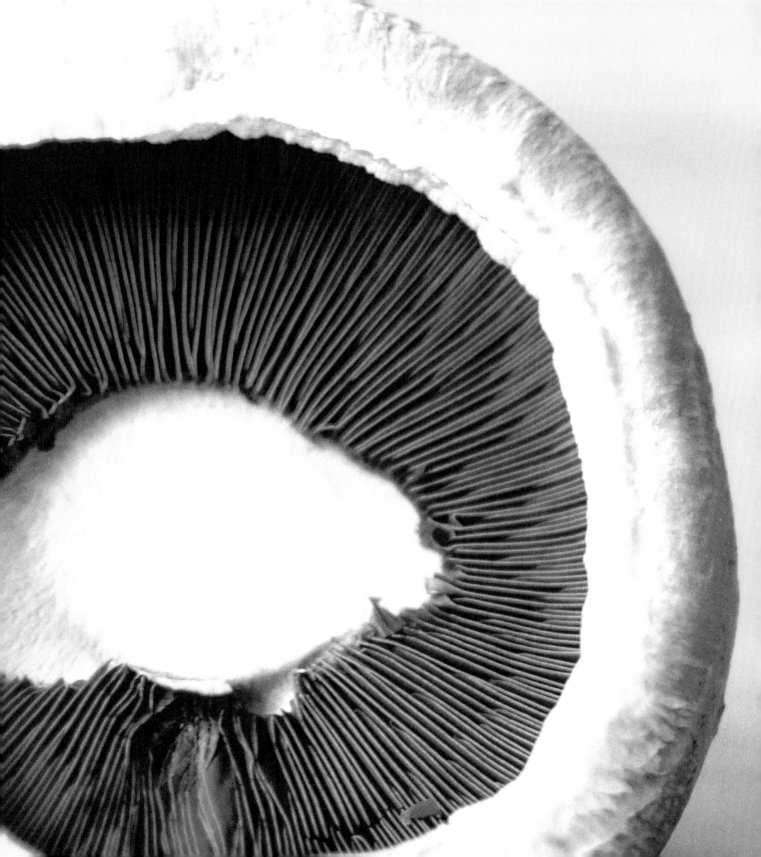

Quinoa Veggie Stir-Fry in Collard Wraps

ingredients

1 cup quinoa

2 cups water

6 eggs

2 tablespoons coconut or sesame oil

2 cloves garlic, peeled and minced

2 tablespoons peeled and minced ginger

6 asparagus stalks, finely chopped

1 red bell pepper, finely chopped

1 medium carrot, finely chopped

4 green onions, chopped

1 cup sliced mushroom (any variety)

1½ cup cashews, whole or chopped

¼ cup low-sodium tamari

¼ cup rice vinegar

6 to 8 large collard greens leaves

Servings: 6

This is another great option for getting more green leafy veggies into the diet. Roll this delicious stir-fry into a collard green wrap. We've witnessed many people learn to love collards in our community cooking classes with this recipe. So, get your wok out and start rolling.

Directions:

1. Add quinoa and water to a saucepan and bring to a boil. Cover and reduce heat to a gentle simmer. Cook for 12 to15 minutes until water is absorbed. Remove from heat, uncover, and let quinoa cool for 5 to 10 minutes.

2. Whisk eggs in a bowl. Heat 1 tablespoon oil in a pan or wok and fry the eggs over medium heat. Set aside in a small bowl.

3. Heat large pan or wok over medium heat and add 1 tablespoon of oil. Add garlic and ginger and sauté for 2 to 3 minutes. Add remainder of vegetables, mushrooms, and cashews. Sauté for an additional 3 to 4 minutes.

4. Gently fold quinoa into the mixture. Add tamari, vinegar, and eggs. Continue stirring until the liquid is absorbed, approximately 3 to 5 minutes.

5. Remove from heat and serve in a bowl or prepare as Collard Wraps.

COLLARD WRAPS:

To blanch collard leaves, begin by cutting off the thick stem just below the bottom of the leaf. Heat water in a medium pot (not boiling). Use tongs to dip each leaf into the hot water for 5 to 10 seconds. The leaf should turn a bright green color and soften. Next, dip leaf into a cold-water bath, or rinse under cold running water. Lay a leaf out flat and spoon stir-fry ingredients onto one end of the leaf. Begin to roll, fold in the sides, and then finish rolling.

Nutrition Facts:

- Cashews are a great source of minerals, as well as monounsaturated fats—the same type of fat found in olives and avocados.

- Mushrooms such as crimini, shitake, portobello, and button can support a healthy immune system. These amazing fungi provide a unique plant-based source of vitamin D as well as numerous other immune-stimulating chemicals.[3] Mushrooms also provide powerful anti-inflammatory effects in the body.[4] Enjoy cooked mushrooms in stir-fries, teas, or soups in order to absorb the most nutrients.

- Quinoa is one of a few whole grains that is a complete protein. It is also high in fiber and contains many minerals such as manganese, magnesium, iron, copper, and phosphorus.

Nut Butter Banana Jam Sandwiches

Peanut butter and jelly sandwiches are loved by many. This recipe reminds us that simple substitutions can really improve the nutritional value of some of our favorite meals. Substituting a whole fruit like banana for sweetened jelly is a healthy alternative. Remember to check your nut butter labels and to avoid added oils, sugars, and preservatives.

ingredients

2 bananas

1 teaspoon cinnamon

8 tablespoons nut butter (peanut, almond, cashew)

8 slices 100% whole grain bread

Serving Size: 4

Directions:

1. Mash bananas in a bowl and add cinnamon.

2. Spread nut butter on bread slices followed by banana jam. Pair up slices. Cut into halves or quarters.

Turkey Avocado Roll-ups

i n g r e d i e n t s

8 slices of turkey
½ cup hummus
1 cup baby spinach
1 medium avocado, thinly sliced
1 cucumber, julienned
4 collard green leaves (optional)

Servings: 4

Directions:

1. Spread a spoonful of hummus on a slice of turkey. Lay a few pieces of spinach flat on the hummus. Place avocado and cucumber at one end of the turkey slice and roll it up. Use a toothpick to hold the roll together, if needed.

2. You may also choose to place a blanched collard green leaf under the turkey slice and follow the directions above.

Tips:

*   To blanch collard leaves, begin by cutting off the thick stem just below the bottom of the leaf. Heat water in a medium pot (not boiling). Use tongs to dip each leaf into the hot water for 5 to 10 seconds. The leaf should turn a bright green color and soften. Next, dip leaf into a cold-water bath, or rinse under cold running water. You are now ready to roll ingredients into your leaf.

Homemade Hummus

Hummus highlights the rich flavor of garbanzo beans while providing a simple, delicious way to include protein, fat, and fiber in your meal. Chopped vegetables of any kind (peppers, carrots, celery, or cucumber) provide an excellent way for adults and children to enjoy hummus.

Directions:

1. Prepare garbanzo beans. (See **Kitchen Skills** for preparing dry beans.) If using canned beans, drain and rinse.

2. Add cooked beans, lemon juice, garlic, tahini, salt, olive oil, and half the water in a blender or food processor. Blend for one minute on medium speed until thoroughly mixed and smooth. Add more water as needed for desired consistency.

Tips:

- Serve immediately with fresh, chopped vegetables. Also consider making **Spring Herb Crackers** to dip in the hummus, or use as a spread for the **Turkey Avocado Roll-ups**. To expand the flavors of the hummus, add fresh greens (spinach or kale), roasted red peppers, jalapeno, or cayenne pepper.

ingredients

1 ½ cups cooked or canned garbanzo beans

¼ cup water

2 tablespoons extra virgin olive oil

1 to 2 teaspoons lemon juice

1 teaspoon tahini (ground sesame seeds)

2 cloves garlic, minced

¼ teaspoon salt

ingredients

1 cup walnuts, chopped

1 cup sunflower seeds (no shell)

1 cup ground flaxseed

1 cup unsweetened shredded coconut

½ cup sesame seeds

1 ½ cups carob chips or dark chocolate chips

1 cup peanut butter or almond butter

½ cup butter or coconut oil

salt, a pinch

Servings: 24 bars

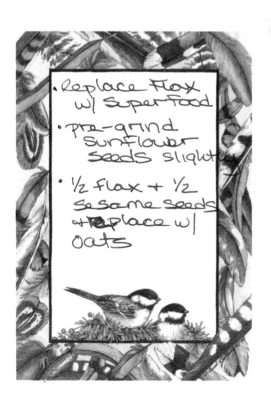

• Replace Flax w/ Superfood

• pre-grind sunflower seeds slightly

• ½ flax + ½ sesame seeds + replace w/ oats

Coco Loco Protein Bars

Directions:

1. Grease a 9 x 13 inch baking pan.

2. Mix together dry ingredients (walnuts, sunflower seeds, sesame seeds, ground flaxseed, and shredded coconut) in a medium bowl.

3. Melt together carob or chocolate chips, nut butter, and butter or coconut oil and a pinch of salt over a double boiler, stirring regularly.

4. Add the dry ingredients to the bowl of melted ingredients and stir until mixed.

5. Press into baking pan. Top with extra shredded coconut or chopped nuts. Chill for 15 minutes in the freezer or one hour in a refrigerator until the bars are solid. Cut into 24 bars.

Tips:

• These bars are very energy-dense and should be eaten in small amounts. Store in the fridge for up to five days.

• If using unsweetened carob chips, chocolate chips, or baker's chocolate, the bars will be bitter. Consider adding ⅓ to ½ cup maple syrup.

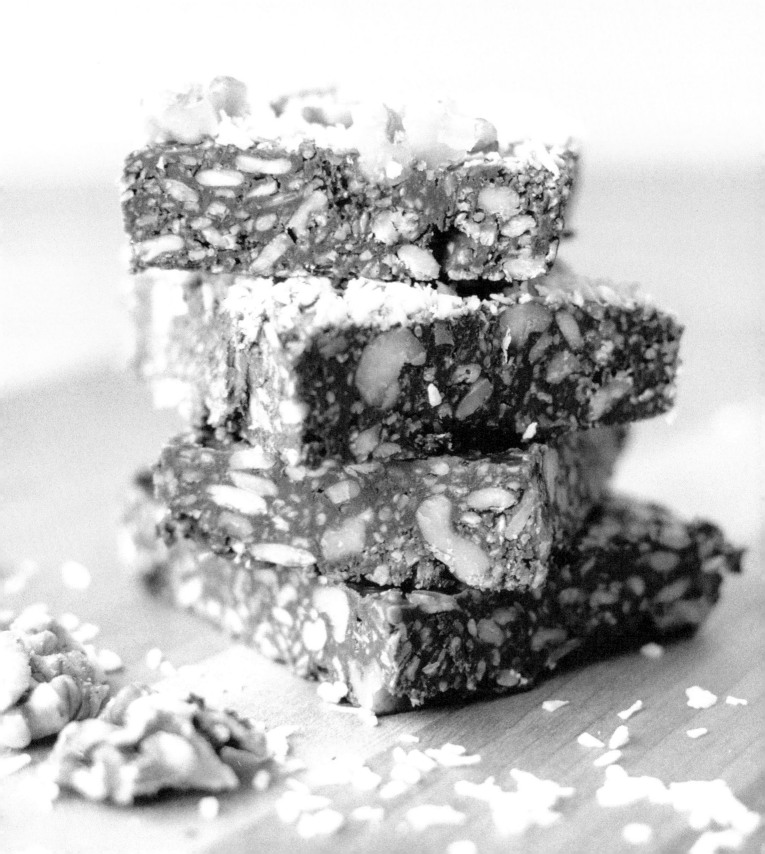

i n g r e d i e n t s

2 cups rolled oats

½ cup raw nuts (slivered almonds, chopped walnuts or hazelnuts)

¼ cup raw seeds (sesame or sunflower)

1 to 2 teaspoons cinnamon

¼ teaspoon salt

¼ cup coconut oil or butter

¼ cup maple syrup

1 teaspoon vanilla extract

¼ cup unsweetened shredded coconut (I used flaked)

¼ cup raisins

Servings: 4 to 6

* Do not cook raisins. Add in once the granola is done. Only cook coconut for the final 5 mins.

Golden Delicious Granola

Store-bought granola can be expensive and full of refined sweeteners and highly processed fats. Save money and enjoy this homemade version using your favorite healthy nuts and seeds. Eat it for a snack, with unsweetened milk or yogurt as a cereal or serve as a topping to chopped fruit. Pay attention to serving size with this sweet treat, since granola contains added sweeteners.

Directions:

1. Preheat the oven to 350°F. **325°**

2. Combine all the dry ingredients, *except* raisins and dried coconut, in one bowl (oats, nuts, seeds, salt, cinnamon).

3. Melt the oil or butter in a saucepan. Add vanilla and maple syrup to the melted oil and mix.

4. Pour the wet ingredients slowly into the dry ingredients and mix thoroughly.

5. Spread the granola on a baking sheet in a thin, even layer and bake for 30 to 40 minutes. Stir the granola every 5 to10 minutes to prevent burning around the edges. After 20 minutes of baking, gently fold in the raisins and dried coconut to mix for the final 10 to 15 minutes of baking. This will prevent the raisins and coconut from browning or being overcooked.

6. Remove from oven and let cool.

7. Leftovers can be stored in an airtight container for up to two weeks.

Tips:

- Experiment with other combinations of nuts, seeds, spices, or dried fruits. Make a double batch for a quick breakfast and for healthy snacking.

Homemade Almond Milk

Store-bought almond milk is hard to find without added sugar and almost always contains the ambiguous *natural flavors*. Avoid unnecessary additives and enjoy a big difference in taste with this homemade almond milk.

Directions:

1. Place the raw almonds in a large bowl and cover with two inches of water. Let the almonds soak for at least six hours, and up to 24 hours. Loosely cover the bowl and keep in the fridge or on your countertop.

2. After soaking, drain the water and rinse the almonds. Add 1 cup soaked almonds and 2 to 3 cups of fresh water (the less water, the more creamy the almond milk will be) to a blender. Add salt and optional ingredients, vanilla and/or cinnamon. Blend on high for 1 to 2 minutes.

3. Once blended, pass the mixture through a fine cheesecloth placed within a strainer over a bowl or pitcher. Press out as much of the almond milk though the cheesecloth as possible.

   Alternatively, you may use a *nut-milk bag*, a fine mesh bag, which can be found at most natural food stores.

Tips:

* Store your homemade almond milk in an airtight container. It will remain fresh in the refrigerator for up to 3 or 4 days. It will settle and separate, but can be shaken to re-mix. The remaining almond pulp in the cheesecloth can be dried in an oven or dehydrated to make almond meal and used for the **Spring Herb Crackers** or added to smoothies for additional nutrition.

ingredients

1 cup raw almonds
3 cups water for soaking
2 to 3 cups water for blending
salt, a pinch
½ teaspoon vanilla extract (optional)
1 teaspoon cinnamon (optional)

Servings: 2 to 3 cups

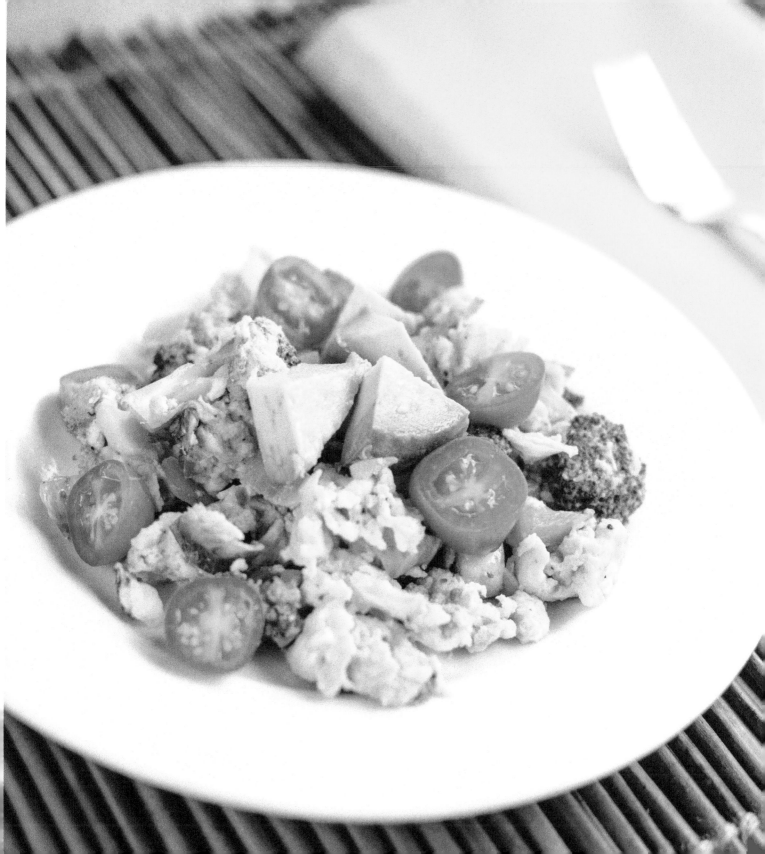

Egg and Veggie Scramble

Finding creative ways to include veggies in a meal can be especially challenging for breakfast. Fear not; here is the savory answer to your morning challenge. With a few minutes of chopping and a few minutes of cooking, you can have a delicious, nutritious scramble to start your day. Use any fresh vegetable in your fridge.

Directions:

1. Chop all veggies into ½-inch pieces.

2. Crack eggs into a mixing bowl and whisk together.

3. Heat oil or butter in a skillet on medium heat and sauté onions until translucent. Add garlic and vegetables and sauté for 3 to 4 minutes, until slightly softened.

4. Lower the heat to low/medium and add the eggs to the skillet. Season with salt and pepper.

5. Stir mixture occasionally, turning the eggs and veggies in the pan. Continue until the eggs are set and no longer runny—approximately 5 minutes.

6. Add optional toppings, avocado and/or tomato and enjoy your morning veggies.

Nutrition Facts:

- Organic, pasture-raised eggs are an excellent source of high quality protein, as well as essential B-vitamins and choline, an important nutrient for healthy brain function.

- Contrary to the common belief that eating cholesterol found in egg yolks will raise *bad* cholesterol levels, this notion has been largely over-exaggerated. Regular consumption of eggs can improve cholesterol levels for many people.[5]

i n g r e d i e n t s

4 cups chopped vegetables (broccoli, bell peppers, mushrooms, zucchini, Brussels sprouts, and greens such as spinach and chard)

8 eggs

2 tablespoons butter or coconut oil

¼ cup diced onion

1 clove garlic, peeled and minced

½ teaspoon salt

¼ teaspoon black pepper

½ avocado, diced (optional)

1 tomato, diced (optional)

Servings: 4

ingredients

*3 cups cooked or canned black
beans*

½ teaspoon cumin

¼ teaspoon cayenne pepper

¼ teaspoon salt

*1 to 1 ½ cups grated cheddar cheese
(optional)*

*8 to 10 ounce bag organic corn or
whole-grain/seed chips*

½ cup diced onion

1 bell pepper, diced

4 kale leaves, finely chopped

1 to 2 tomatoes, diced

Servings: 4 to 6

Rainbow Nachos

Rainbow Nachos are a fun and delicious way to get vegetables into the diet and make nachos a quick and healthy meal choice.

Directions:

1. Pre-heat the oven to 375°F.

2. If using canned beans, drain and rinse. In a bowl, mix beans with cumin, cayenne pepper, and salt.

3. Grate the cheese.

4. Spread chips out on a baking sheet. Layer first with beans. Then, add the chopped onions, bell pepper, kale, and tomatoes. Top with grated cheese.

5. Place in oven and bake for approximately 10 minutes until the cheese is melted.

6. Top with guacamole, chopped cilantro, diced tomatoes, or fresh salsa.

Tips:

- Add an additional layer to your nachos of cooked and diced chicken breast (a Rotisserie chicken works great) or cooked ground beef, chicken, or turkey for additional protein and delicious flavor.

Nutrition Facts:

- Black beans are a rich source of fiber—1 cup contains about 15 grams of fiber and 15 grams of protein.

  Black beans are also high in folate. Folate is an important B vitamin that is protective against cardiovascular disease.

- Kale is an excellent source of beta-carotene (precursor to vitamin A) and vitamin K, and a good source of folate. In addition, kale is a great way to include a plant-based source of calcium in your diet.

- Tomatoes are rich in immune-supporting vitamin C and in the anti-oxidant lycopene, which protects our eyes and the prostate gland in men. Tomatoes are often excluded in many anti-inflammatory diets because of anecdotal evidence that shows a worsening of osteoarthritis symptoms for some individuals. While some people may have sensitivities to this plant and should avoid it, we are big fans of the amazing colors and protective plant compounds that tomatoes bring to many meals.

Guacamole

Directions:

1. Peel the avocados, remove the pit and mash with a fork or potato masher to a smooth texture. Mix in onions, garlic, tomato, cilantro, lime juice, salt and jalapeno (optional).

2. Serve immediately.

Tips:

- Serve with **Rainbow Nachos**, **Egg and Veggie Scramble** or with **Refried Beans and Rice**.

Nutrition Facts:

- Most of us think of bananas as the potassium power-house. Move over banana, here comes avocado! One medium banana contains 422 mg of potassium while one medium avocado contains up to 700 mg of potassium and 10 grams of fiber! Potassium is a critical mineral for healthy heart function. Our bodies work best with a potassium-to-sodium ratio of greater than two parts potassium to one part sodium. A lower ratio puts us at risk for heart disease. In the Standard American Diet, people generally are over-consuming sodium and under-consuming potassium. Reducing added salt in the diet from processed foods and

ingredients

2 to 3 ripe avocados

2 tablespoons finely diced red onion

1 clove garlic, peeled and minced

1 tomato, diced

¼ cup finely chopped cilantro

2 tablespoons lime juice

¼ to ½ teaspoon salt

1 jalapeno, minced (optional)

Servings: 4 to 6

ingredients

eating fresh fruits and vegetables will improve your potassium to sodium ratio.

Avocados also provide a rich source of monounsaturated fats, which help the body to absorb other fat-soluble vitamins such as vitamins A, D, E, and K.

Vegetable Broth

Vegetable broth delivers vitamins and minerals as well as delicious flavor to many recipes. The wonderful thing about making veggie broth is that you can use any vegetables available, even your veggie scraps from other recipes. Save your scraps from chopped carrots, bell pepper, mushrooms, fennel, celery, onion skins, and stems and leaves from all dark green leafy veggies. Freeze the scraps and when you have saved enough, make a broth. Use the directions below as a guideline.

1 tablespoon coconut oil

1 onion, diced

8 cloves garlic, peeled and minced

2 carrots, chopped

2 stalks celery, including leaves, chopped

4 sprigs fresh rosemary

2 sprigs fresh thyme

2 bay leaves

1 teaspoon salt (optional)

8 cups water

2 cups additional vegetable scraps (optional)

Servings: Makes 8 cups

Directions:

1. Chop all vegetables into 1-inch or smaller pieces.

2. Heat a large pot over medium heat and add oil. Add onion and sauté until translucent, about 3 to 5 minutes.

3. Add garlic, carrots, and celery. Sauté for another 3 to 5 minutes until softened.

4. Add water, herbs, and additional vegetables and bring to a boil. Add salt if desired. Lower heat and simmer, uncovered, for at least 60 minutes. You can strain the vegetables or blend all ingredients together with an immersion blender, creating a thicker broth.

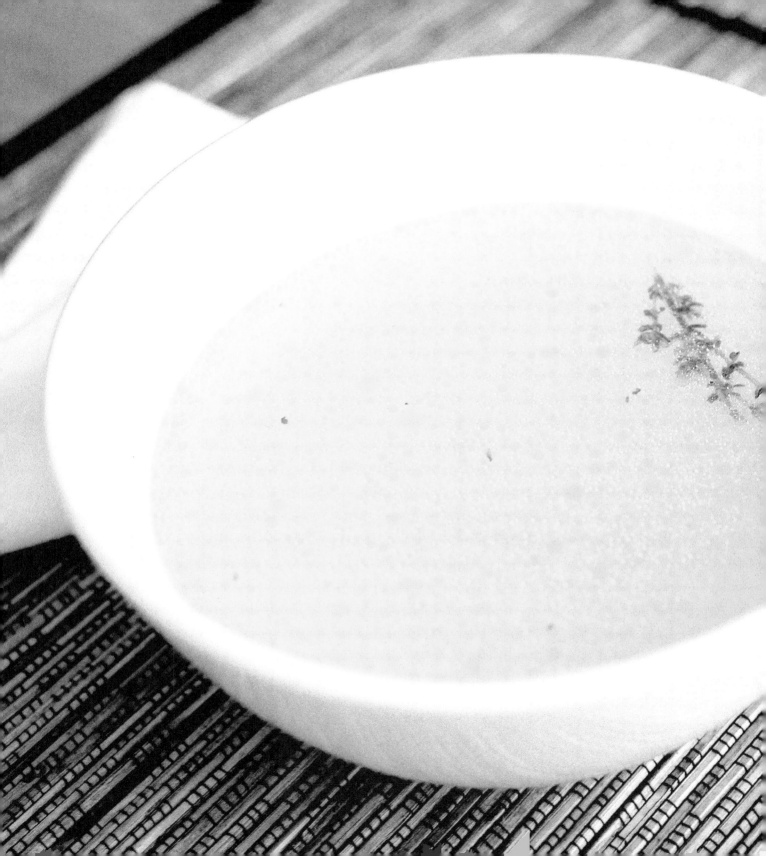

Basic Bone Broth

ingredients

4 pounds bones from organic,
    pasture-raised chicken, cow,
    lamb, or turkey
1 carrot, diced
1 onion, diced
4 cloves garlic, peeled and minced
2 tablespoons apple cider vinegar
16 cups water (equal to one gallon)

The health benefits of nutrient-dense bone broth are numerous! Bone broth promotes strong bones and healthy hair because of the high mineral content and gelatin. It contains amino acids like cysteine and arginine that support a healthy immune response. Bone broth provides abundant and easily absorbable vitamins and minerals, which can be helpful to those who are sick or are healing a troubled gut. This broth also contains important building blocks for chondroitin sulphate and glucosamine for healthy joints. While some planning is required, preparing bone broth at home is an investment in your health.

Directions:

1. Add all ingredients in a large stockpot and simmer on low heat for at least 8 to 12 hours.
2. Occasionally skim foam that collects on the surface.
3. After 8 to 12 hours, strain the bones and vegetables from the liquid. Enjoy the bone broth by itself or use it as a base for other soups.

Tips:

*   The broth can be stored in the refrigerator for three days or in the freezer for three months.

Nutrition Facts:

*   The addition of vinegar allows for the extraction of the healthy minerals and amino acids from the bones.

SPRING AND SUMMER

i n g r e d i e n t s

*2 tablespoons olive oil, butter, or
    coconut oil*

1 yellow onion, diced

2 stalks celery, finely diced

2 carrots, finely diced

5 cloves garlic, peeled and minced

2 cups red lentils

8 cups low-sodium vegetable broth

1 cup fresh parsley, chopped

1 cup fresh basil, chopped

5 cups spinach, finely chopped

½ cup lemon juice

1 teaspoon salt

Servings: 6 to 8

Spring Lentil Soup

Soup is a delicious way to add more greens to the diet. Lentils provide an excellent, plant-based protein and have a short cooking time. In springtime, this herb-rich lentil soup pairs wonderfully with **Spring Herb Crackers**.

Directions:

1. Heat a large stockpot over medium heat and add oil or butter. Add onions and sauté for 3 to 4 minutes. Then add celery, carrots, and garlic. Sauté for an additional 3 to 4 minutes.

2. Rinse and drain red lentils and add to pot along with the broth. Bring to a boil and cover. Reduce heat and simmer for 20 to 25 minutes, until lentils are soft and thoroughly cooked.

3. Remove stockpot from heat and add parsley, basil, spinach, lemon juice, and salt. Stir until well combined and serve.

Spring Herb Crackers

These simple, savory gluten-free crackers are FAME favorites.

Directions:

1. Preheat oven to 350°F.
2. Combine almond meal, salt, and fresh chopped herbs in a bowl.
3. Whisk together melted oil or butter and egg in a separate bowl.
4. Stir wet ingredients into almond meal mixture until thoroughly combined.
5. Roll the dough into a ball. On a baking sheet, press dough between two sheets of parchment paper to $1/8$ to $1/4$ inch thickness. Use a rolling pin, if available.
6. Remove top piece of parchment paper.
7. Cut dough into 2-inch squares or other desired shape with a knife or pizza cutter.
8. Bake for 9 to 14 minutes, until lightly golden. Watch carefully.
9. Let crackers cool on baking sheet for 10 minutes, then serve.

ingredients

1¾ cups almond meal
½ teaspoon salt
2 tablespoons finely chopped fresh rosemary or thyme, without the stem
1 teaspoon finely chopped fennel seed (optional)
1 tablespoon coconut oil or butter
1 egg

Servings: Makes 24 crackers

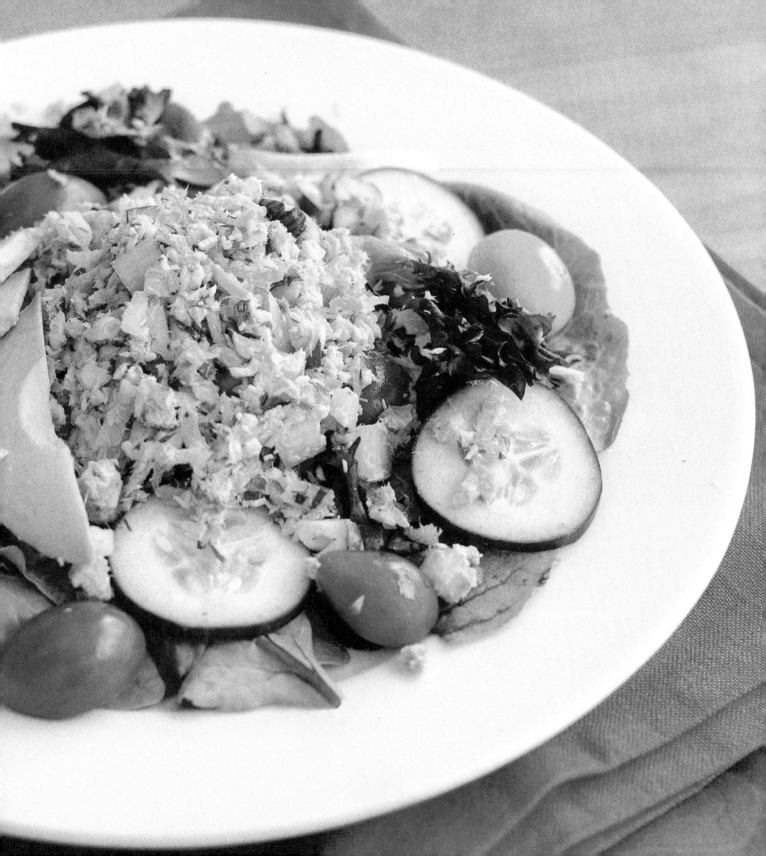

Hearty Salmon Salad

This colorful, nutrient-packed, cold salad is a perfect meal for a warm day or for a potluck gathering. Wild salmon, fresh veggies, herbs, and a zesty dressing make this one of the most popular meals in our community cooking classes. We also make and enjoy a naturally sweet treat with fresh berries and spiced coconut milk. **Coconut Berry Bliss** is a great alternative to typical desserts with high amounts of sugar and refined carbohydrates.

Directions:

1. In a large bowl, add salmon and use a fork to pull the fish apart.

2. Add olive oil, carrots, celery, onion, lemon juice, dill, tarragon, and parsley to the bowl and mix. Set aside.

3. In a large salad bowl, add lettuce or mixed greens with chopped cucumbers, tomatoes, and hazelnuts.

4. Place salmon salad mixture on top of green salad. Drizzle dressing of choice onto salad and salmon. See recipe for **Basic Vinaigrette Dressing**. Serve immediately.

Tips:

- Use canned salmon or leftover baked or grilled salmon. Small bones found in canned salmon can be eaten as they are an excellent food source of calcium. The salmon salad can be stored for 3 to 4 days in the refrigerator. It makes a great *to-go* lunch.

Nutrition Facts:

- Omega-3 fatty acids are essential fatty acids that must be obtained from the diet. Omega-3 fatty acids help to reduce inflammation and to support a healthy heart and cognitive function, including memory.[6] Rich sources of omega-3 fatty acids are found in salmon, tuna, algae, krill, cod, ground flax and chia seeds, and walnuts.

ingredients

SALMON SALAD:

12 to 18 ounces canned or cooked wild-caught salmon (3 oz. per person)
5 tablespoons extra virgin olive oil
1 carrot, finely grated
2 stalks celery, finely diced
½ medium red onion, finely diced
¼ to ½ cup lemon juice
1 teaspoon finely chopped fresh dill,
1 teaspoon finely chopped fresh tarragon
2 tablespoons finely chopped fresh parsley

GREEN SALAD:

1 head red or green leaf lettuce, chopped, or 6 to 8 cups mixed greens
1 cucumber, sliced
2 tomatoes, sliced or 1 cup cherry tomatoes
1 cup hazelnuts, chopped

Servings: 4 to 6

i n g r e d i e n t s

- Eating salmon regularly can support healthy cholesterol levels, regulation of heart rhythm, and improved health outcomes in those with heart disease.[7] Choose wild Alaskan or Pacific salmon rather than farmed salmon, due to the concern of environmental toxicity in farmed salmon.[8]

Basic Vinaigrette Dressing

½ cup extra virgin olive oil

¼ cup vinegar (balsamic, apple cider)

1 teaspoon maple syrup or raw honey

1 teaspoon mustard

¼ teaspoon salt or to taste

⅛ teaspoon ground black pepper

1 tablespoon finely chopped fresh or
    dried herbs (parsley, tarragon, dill)

Directions:

Combine ingredients in small bowl and whisk together.

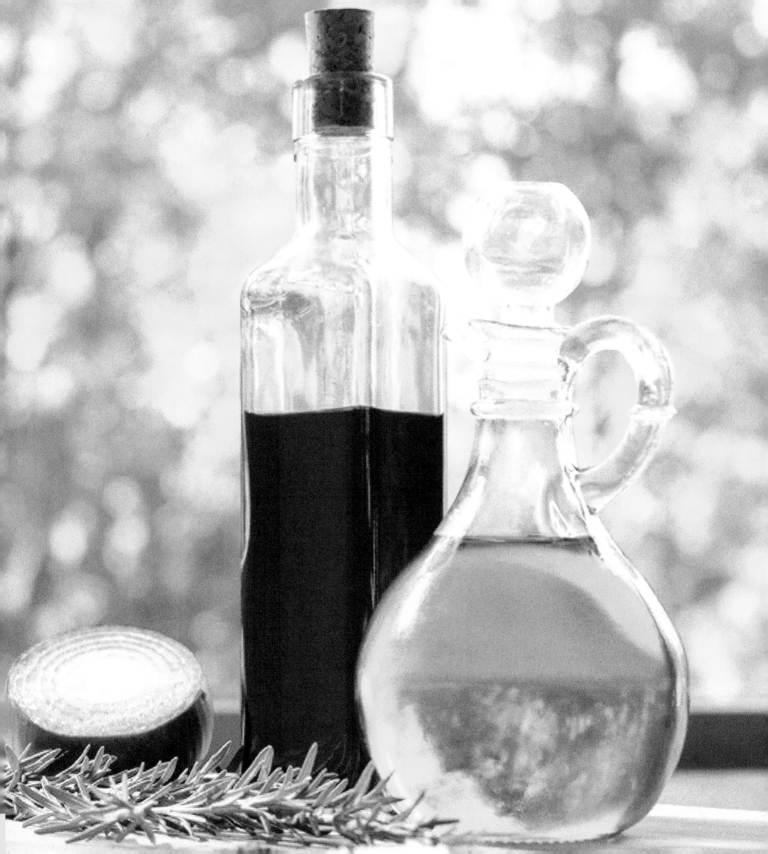

ingredients

1 cup full-fat canned coconut milk

1 tablespoon maple syrup

½ teaspoon cinnamon

⅛ teaspoon salt

½ teaspoon vanilla

4 cups fresh or frozen berries (raspberries, blueberries, strawberries)

4 tablespoons ground flaxseed

4 tablespoons chopped nuts (optional)

Servings: 4

Coconut Berry Bliss

Directions:

1. Mix coconut milk with maple syrup, cinnamon, salt, and vanilla in small bowl. For a thicker version, remove and use only the cream from the top of the canned coconut milk.

2. Place one cup of berries into each of four small bowls. Add ¼ cup of coconut mixture plus 1 tablespoon of ground flaxseed and 1 tablespoon chopped nuts (optional) on top of each bowl of fruit. Serve immediately.

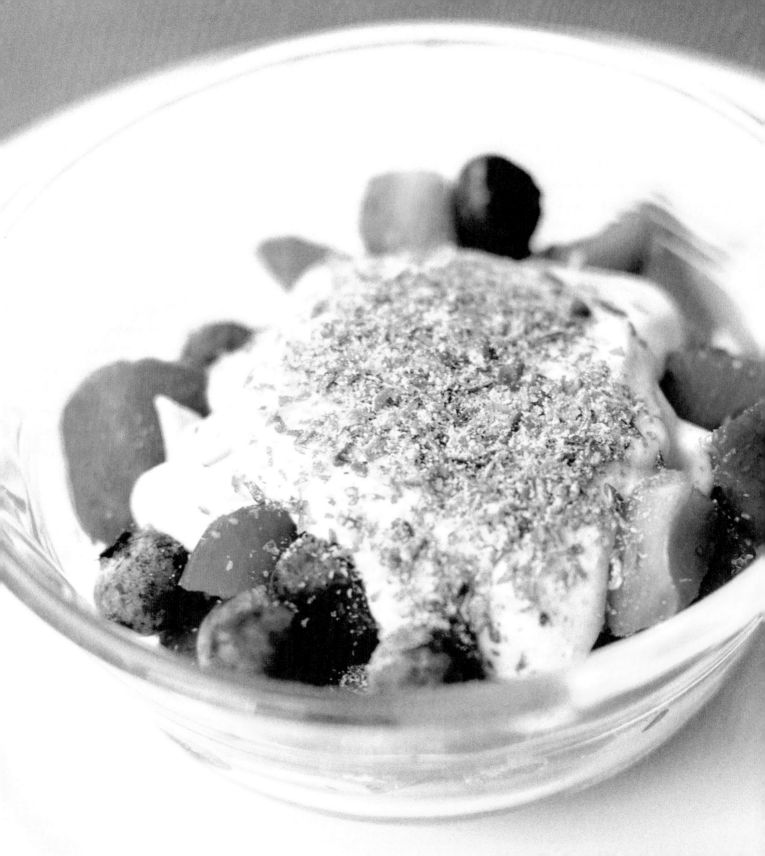

ingredients

3 cups cooked or canned garbanzo
    or white beans
1 cup sliced and quartered zucchini
1 tomato, diced
1 clove garlic, peeled and minced
½ cup finely copped fresh basil
    leaves
2 tablespoons finely chopped fresh
    oregano, without stems
2 tablespoons finely chopped fresh
    parsley
½ teaspoon salt
¼ teaspoon black pepper

DRESSING INGREDIENTS:
½ cup extra virgin olive oil
¼ cup apple cider vinegar
1 clove garlic, peeled and minced
1 teaspoon finely chopped fresh
    herbs, (oregano, parley, basil, or
    combination)
1 teaspoon finely diced onion
1 teaspoon Dijon mustard
¼ teaspoon salt
$1/8$ teaspoon black pepper

Servings: 6

Garden-fresh Summer Squash Salad

If you have a garden, you will likely be able to supply most of the ingredients for this colorful, herb-filled recipe. Enjoy the inspiring scents provided by the spring herbs. We often choose to create this dish during the Healthy Digestion workshop because it truly inspires mindfulness with your meal.

Directions for salad:

1. In a medium bowl, combine beans, zucchini, tomato, garlic, basil, oregano, and parsley. Add salt and pepper. Toss gently.

2. Combine all dressing ingredients in bowl and wisk together.

3. Add dressing to the salad mixture and mix. Marinate salad for at least 30 minutes in the refrigerator before serving. Serve over **Lemon Rice**.

Lemon Rice

Refresh your brown rice with lemon and herbs!

Directions:

1. Combine broth, coconut oil, and rice into medium saucepan.

2. Bring to a boil, then reduce heat.

3. Cover pot and allow to simmer for 40 to 45 minutes, or until liquid is absorbed.

4. Remove from heat. Stir in lemon juice and basil. Fluff with a fork before serving.

Tips:

- Substitute chicken broth or water to cook the rice.

ingredients

2½ cups low-sodium vegetable broth

2 teaspoons butter or coconut oil

1 cup brown rice

¼ cup lemon juice

1 teaspoon finely chopped fresh basil

Servings: 4

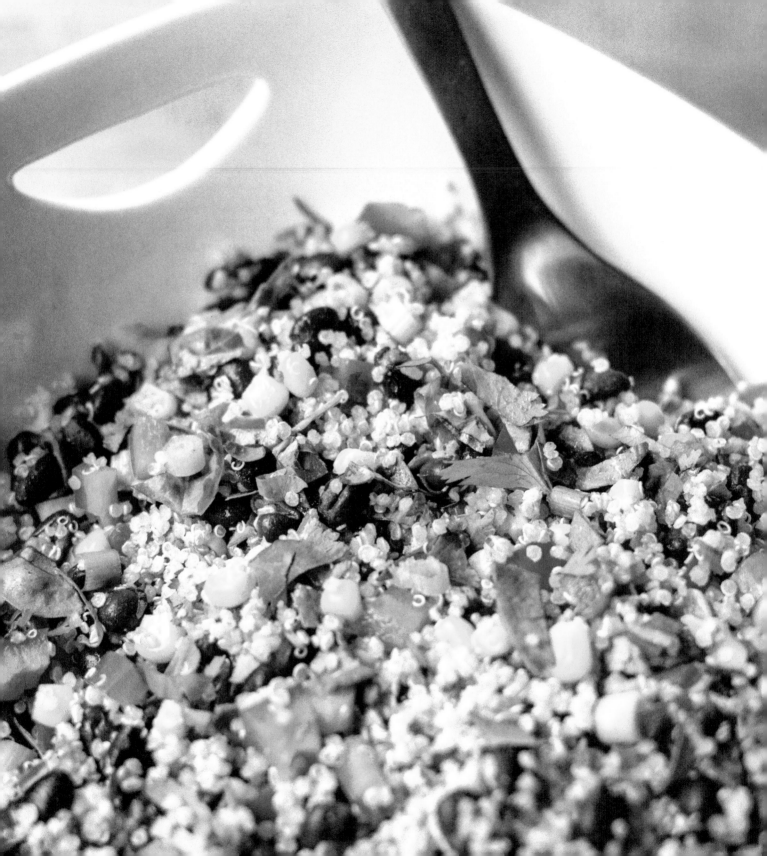

Rainbow Quinoa Salad

This is a colorful recipe to add to your cooking repertoire, and it has an abundance of flavor! Colorful meals ensure you are consuming a wide range of vitamins, minerals, and antioxidants. This quinoa salad can be served warm or cold, enjoyed in a collard green wrap, or served as a taco or burrito filling.

Directions:

1. To prepare the quinoa: Bring two cups of water to a boil in a medium saucepan. Add 1 cup quinoa and return to a boil. Reduce heat to simmer, cover, and cook for 12 to 15 minutes, until water is absorbed. Remove from heat. Add chopped spinach on top of quinoa, cover with a lid, and steam for 3 minutes. Let the quinoa sit for an additional five minutes and then fluff with a fork.

2. If using canned beans, drain and rinse. While quinoa is cooking, mix the black beans, corn, bell pepper, tomatoes, green onion, and cilantro in a separate bowl and gently stir.

3. In a separate bowl, whisk together the dressing ingredients.

4. Fold the quinoa into the bean mixture. Slowly add the dressing. Stir until mixed well.

5. Add diced avocado and enjoy.

Nutrition Facts:

• Quinoa adds a plant-based, complete protein to the recipe. The beans add protein and fiber. Tomatoes are a excellent source of vitamin C and the antioxidant, lycopene.

i n g r e d i e n t s

1 cup quinoa (red or white)

2 cups water

2 cups finely chopped spinach

2 to 3 cups cooked or canned black beans

1 cup frozen corn, thawed

1 red or orange bell pepper, diced

2 medium tomatoes, diced

5 green onions, chopped

¼ cup chopped cilantro

1 avocado, diced

DRESSING INGREDIENTS:

½ cup extra virgin olive oil

¼ cup apple cider vinegar

¼ cup lime juice

1 teaspoon salt

1 teaspoon cumin

⅛ teaspoon chili powder

black pepper to taste

Servings: 4 to 6

ingredients

¾ pound (1 bunch) dark green leafy
greens (rainbow chard, mustard
greens, dandelion greens, kale)
2 tablespoons healthy fat (butter,
coconut oil, lard, tallow)
6 cloves garlic, finely chopped
3 teaspoons diced yellow onion
2 tablespoons apple cider vinegar

Sautéed Seasonal Greens

Simply sautéing dark green leafy veggies with a healthy fat, such as butter, coconut oil, or animal fats, such as lard and tallow, is a great way to enjoy them. The recipe below can be adapted to include your favorite spices.

Directions:

1. Chop or tear greens into smaller pieces. Remove thick stems if present.

2. Heat pan over medium heat and add healthy fat of your choosing.

3. Add onion and garlic and sauté for 2 to 3 minutes.

4. Add the greens and gently stir until the leaves are wilted, but still a bright green color.

5. Add apple cider vinegar and enjoy.

Nutrition Facts:

- Green leaves are a good source of beta-carotene, a precursor to vitamin A, and many minerals including calcium. Green leaves provide fiber and flavonoids, which are color components of food that aid in protecting the body against toxins.

Summer Tomato Avocado Soup

A salad or side dish that includes a healthy source of protein will help balance the healthy fats found in this refreshing summer soup.

Directions:

1. Add diced tomato, red onion, cucumber, red pepper, garlic, olive oil, vinegar, and all spices into a blender, and blend until creamy.
2. Chill for one hour in the refrigerator.
3. Serve soup in a bowl with diced avocado, cilantro, and a dollop of sour cream or plain yogurt (optional) and enjoy.

i n g r e d i e n t s

4 large tomatoes, diced
½ red onion, diced
½ cucumber, diced
½ red pepper, diced
1 clove garlic, peeled and minced
2 tablespoon extra virgin olive oil
1 tablespoon apple cider vinegar
¾ teaspoon salt
½ teaspoon cumin
⅛ teaspoon cayenne (optional)
3 avocados, diced
2 tablespoons chopped cilantro
Sour cream or plain yogurt (optional)

Servings: 6

ingredients

8 cups chopped dark green salad
    leaves (Romaine, green or red
    lettuce, mixed greens, spinach)

12 ounces cooked turkey, chicken,
    fish, or steak

2 eggs, hard-boiled

1 cucumber, diced

2 tomatoes, diced

½ cup sunflower seeds

1 carrot, finely chopped

1 avocado, sliced

BASIC VINAIGRETTE DRESSING:

½ cup extra virgin olive oil

¼ cup vinegar (balsamic or apple
    cider)

1 teaspoon raw honey

1 teaspoon mustard

¼ teaspoon salt

⅛ teaspoon black pepper

Servings: 4

Basic Green Salad with Protein

Add any healthy source of protein to this salad for a balanced meal
including chicken, fish, turkey, or steak. A simple salad and leftover
cooked meat or poultry makes for a quick, healthy dinner or lunch.
The dressing can be made ahead of time and used throughout the
week.

Directions:

1. Chop or tear green leaves into small pieces. Chop vegetables
   into 1-inch cubes. Slice hard-boiled eggs. Chop meat, fish, or
   poultry into small pieces. Add all ingredients into a large salad
   bowl.

2. Whisk dressing ingredients together.

3. Drizzle dressing on the salad and enjoy.

Tips:

- To hard-boil eggs, place 6 eggs in a single layer at the bottom
  of a saucepan. Cover with 2 inches of cold water. Heat the pot
  on high heat and bring the water to a full rolling boil for 1 to
  2 minutes. Turn off the heat, keep the pan on the hot burner,
  and let sit for 10 to 12 minutes. Carefully pour off the hot water
  from the pan and run very cold water over the eggs to cool them
  quickly and stop them from cooking further. Crack and peel
  away shells of 2 eggs for recipe and store the extra hard boiled
  eggs in a covered container in the refrigerator. Eat as a healthy
  snack within 5 days.

Nutrition Facts:

- The protein, fat, and fiber found in this basic green salad with
  added protein of your choice provide slow fuel to the body
  to support healthy blood sugar regulation as well as building
  blocks for neurotransmitters in the brain. Poultry is a great
  source of protein and tryptophan. Tryptophan is an amino acid
  precursor to the *feel good* neurotransmitter, serotonin.

FALL AND WINTER

ingredients

1 tablespoon coconut oil or butter
½ yellow onion, diced
4 cloves garlic, peeled and minced
1 red pepper, diced
4 cups diced tomato, with liquid, or
    1 can (32 ounces) diced toma-
    toes
4 cups cooked or canned beans
    (kidney, black, pinto or combi-
    nation)
1 cup frozen corn
1 cup low-sodium vegetable or
    chicken broth
1 teaspoon salt
½ teaspoon black pepper
2 tablespoons cumin
2 tablespoon chili powder
⅛ teaspoon cayenne pepper
⅛ teaspoon cinnamon
1 ½ cups finely chopped spinach or
    kale

TOPPINGS:
2 avocados, diced
½ cup chopped fresh cilantro

Serving size: 8

Bean and Veggie Chili

This recipe is a healthy twist on a fall and winter comfort food. It's a wholesome, one pot meal and is great to make in double batches to freeze. Use this recipe to avoid the excessive sodium, artificial flavors, and poor quality meat found in canned chili. Any veggies can be added, especially dark green leafy greens. Add ground turkey, chicken, or beef for an extra protein punch. The **Easy Cornbread** recipe accompanies this recipe well.

Directions:

1. Heat large pot over medium heat and add oil. Sauté onions until translucent, about 3-5 minutes.
2. Add garlic and red pepper and sauté for additional 3 minutes.
3. Add diced tomato, beans, corn, and vegetable or chicken broth. Add spices and bring to a boil.
4. Reduce heat and simmer for 20-30 minutes. Add additional broth if needed.
5. Add the spinach in the last 5 minutes of cooking.
6. Top each bowl of chili with chopped cilantro and diced avocado.

Tips:

- If using canned tomatoes or beans, look for these items in glass jars or in cans or packaging that is BPA-free. Check the bulk section of grocery stores for a premixed chili blend, which will often contain cumin, chili pepper, garlic powder, oregano, coriander, cloves, and allspice.

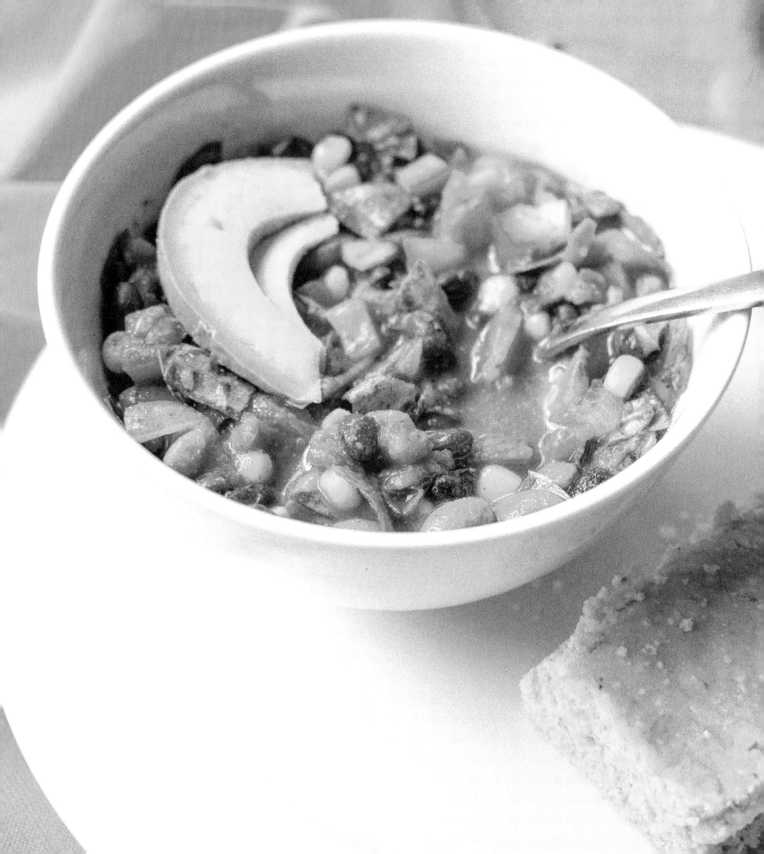

Easy Cornbread

ingredients

1 ½ cups cornmeal, medium or fine
    grind
1 ½ cups brown rice flour
1 teaspoon baking powder
½ teaspoon baking soda
1 teaspoon salt
1 ½ cups milk (unsweetened
    almond, coconut milk, or dairy)
3 tablespoons maple syrup
2 eggs
½ cup coconut oil or butter, melted

Servings: 16

Directions:

1. Preheat oven to 375°F.

2. Grease a 9 x 13 inch baking pan.

3. In a large bowl, mix together the cornmeal, brown rice flour, baking powder, baking soda, and salt.

4. In a second bowl, whisk together the milk, maple syrup, eggs, and melted oil or butter.

5. Add the dry ingredients to the wet ingredients and stir—just until combined.

6. Pour batter into pan and bake until golden brown, 25 to 30 minutes. A toothpick inserted in the middle should come out clean. Serve while warm.

Tips:

*   If you are avoiding eggs, consider the following egg substitutions for baking:

    1 egg = ¼ cup unsweetened applesauce = 1 tablespoon ground flaxseed with ¼ cup hot water; let sit for 5 minutes to create a gelatinous consistency.

Ginger Tempeh Stir Fry with Quinoa

The sesame oil, ginger, and garlic in this dish provide a warming meal. Tamari is a fermented, gluten-free soy sauce, making it a ideal option for those avoiding wheat in the diet. This is a terrific recipe with which to practice creating your healthy FAME plate with appropriate portion sizes.

Directions:

1. Add the dressing ingredients- sesame oil, rice vinegar, tamari, raw honey or maple syrup, ginger root, and garlic to a small bowl and whisk.

2. Prepare the tempeh: Cut the tempeh into 2-inch cubes, or slice into ½ inch strips. Marinate the tempeh in ½ cup of the ginger tamari dressing for 10 to 15 minutes prior to sautéing.

3. While the tempeh is marinating, prepare the quinoa. Bring three cups of water to a boil in a medium saucepan. Add 1 ½ cup quinoa and return to a boil. Reduce heat to simmer, cover, and cook for 12 to 15 minutes, until water is absorbed. Remove from heat. Let the quinoa sit for five minutes and then fluff with a fork.

4. Dice the vegetables and cut the broccoli into florets. Heat 2 tablespoons of sesame oil over medium heat in a large frying pan or wok and add the vegetables. Pour remaining dressing onto vegetables and cook for 5 to 10 minutes until vegetables are softened but still brightly color. Add cashews to the mix for the last few minutes.

5. In a large skillet, add the tempeh with marinade sauce and cook it for 5 to 10 minutes, turning frequently, until the tempeh is lightly browned.

6. Create a healthy FAME plate: Serve 1 to 2 cups of cooked vegetables on half of the plate. Place ½ cup of quinoa on one quarter of the plate. Add 3 ounce serving of tempeh on one quarter of the plate.

12 ounces organic tempeh
3 cups water
1½ cup quinoa
2 tablespoons sesame oil
6 to 8 cups chopped vegetables, including onion, broccoli, carrots, celery, bok choy, snow peas, and/or cabbage
¾ cup of cashews

Ginger Tamari Dressing
½ cup sesame oil
¼ cup rice vinegar
¼ cup low-sodium tamari
1 tablespoon maple syrup or raw honey
1 teaspoon peeled and minced ginger root
1 clove garlic, peeled and minced

Servings: 4 to 6

Nutrition Facts:

- If consuming soy, we recommend choosing minimally processed, fermented, non-genetically modified (non-GMO), organic soy, which includes tempeh, miso, tamari, and natto. The fermentation of the soybeans helps decrease some of the plant-based chemicals that can affect hormones and digestion. These include goitrogens (which inhibit thyroid function), phytic acid (which blocks nutrient absorption) and phytoestrogens (which influence estrogen activity in the body).

- Soybeans provide a complete plant-based protein. Studies have shown soy to beneficially impact cholesterol levels and to contribute a good source of fiber to the diet.[9]

- Broccoli is a cruciferous vegetable that is high in carotenoids and antioxidants, which can be protective against cancer and inflammation.[10] It is an excellent source of vitamin C, A, K, folate, calcium, and fiber.

- Cashew nuts are a rich source of monounsaturated fats, like olive oil and avocados. This healthy fat, along with the presence of antioxidants, fiber, phytosterols, magnesium, and folate, all contribute to the cashew nut's ability to reduce the risk of heart disease. Eating nuts at least five times a week has been shown to reduce the risk of heart disease and diabetes by 20% to 50%![11] Including nuts with a meal also assists with balanced blood sugar by slowing digestion.

Black-eyed Peas and Collard Greens Soup

Black-eyed peas and collard greens are a traditional southern United States dish. Collards are often boiled over a long period of time with a ham hock and the black-eyed peas are served separately. This variation is a soup that brings together the greens and the beans with extra veggies and can save you some time in the kitchen. The **Sweet Potato Cornbread** recipe makes a great side dish for this soup.

Directions:

1. Heat a large pot over medium heat and add oil or butter. Add onion and sauté until translucent, about 3 to 5 minutes.

2. Add garlic, carrots, and celery. Sauté for another 3 to 5 minutes until softened.

3. Add the cooked black-eyed peas, broth, and seasonings- cumin, chili powder, salt, pepper, cayenne (optional). Bring to a boil. Reduce heat and simmer for about 20 minutes.

4. Add the chopped collard greens and simmer 10 more minutes.

5. Remove from heat and enjoy immediately.

Tips:

- Soups, in general, make great leftovers. Make a double batch and enjoy throughout the week.

3 tablespoons coconut oil, butter or animal fat (lard, tallow)

1 yellow onion, chopped

4 cloves garlic, peeled and minced

6 stalks celery, chopped

4 carrots, chopped

3 cups cooked or canned black-eyed peas

5 to 6 cups low-sodium vegetable broth

2 teaspoons cumin

1 teaspoon chili powder

1 teaspoon salt

½ teaspoon black pepper

⅛ teaspoon cayenne pepper (optional)

¾ pound (1 bunch) collard greens, stems removed, finely chopped

Serving size: 6 to 8

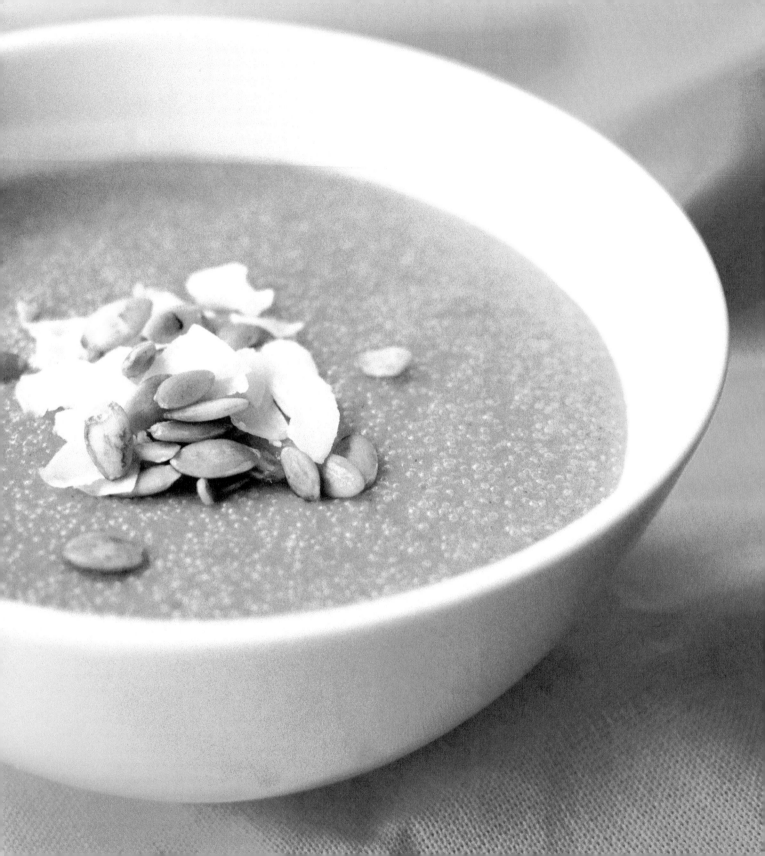

Pumpkin Pie Amaranth Porridge

Amaranth, like quinoa, provides a complete, plant-based protein. Amaranth is actually a very tiny seed that dates back 8,000 years as a traditional staple grain of the Aztecs in Mexico. This warming, savory porridge is rich in protein and healthy fat, not to mention sweet spices. What a wonderful way to start the day. We love the addition of pumpkin puree and seeds to add flavor and texture to the porridge.

Directions:

1. Combine amaranth with water in medium pot and bring to a boil. Reduce heat to simmer, cover, and cook for 20 to 25 minutes, until water is absorbed.

2. Add the pumpkin puree, coconut milk, salt, spices, and vanilla and stir. Then, turn the heat off. Let the porridge sit and thicken for a few minutes with the lid on.

3. Sweeten with maple syrup if desired. Drizzle with extra coconut milk. Sprinkle with ground pumpkin seeds and coconut flakes.

Tips:

* Sweet potato puree can be substituted for the pumpkin.

* Use a pre-blended "pumpkin pie spice" puree to simplify the recipe.

* To modify this recipe for the summer season, cook the amaranth with the water and coconut milk. After removing from the heat, add fresh berries and let porridge sit for 5 to 10 minutes. Add maple syrup along with cinnamon or ginger to sweeten as desired.

ingredients

1 cup amaranth

2½ cups water

1½ cups full-fat canned coconut milk

¾ cup pureed pumpkin (fresh or canned)

½ teaspoon salt

½ teaspoon cinnamon

¼ teaspoon ginger, dried

¼ teaspoon nutmeg

$\frac{1}{8}$ teaspoon ground cloves

1 teaspoon vanilla extract

2 tablespoons maple syrup (optional)

4 tablespoons pumpkin seeds (optional)

¾ cup coconut flakes (optional)

Servings: 4 to 6

Sweet Potato Cornbread

i n g r e d i e n t s

1 cup pureed or mashed sweet
    potato

1½ cups cornmeal, fine or medium-
    grind

1½ cups brown rice flour

1 teaspoons baking powder

½ teaspoon baking soda

½ teaspoon salt

1 egg

¼ cup maple syrup

¹/₃ cup coconut oil or butter, melted

Servings: Makes 24 pieces

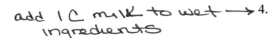
add 1 C milk to wet →
    ingredients

Sweet potato cornbread is a delicious and sweet side dish. We recommend using the brightly colored orange sweet potatoes (often labeled as jewel or garnet yams) to make a beautiful cornbread that is also high in antioxidants, specifically beta-carotene. Make this recipe a gluten-free cornbread by choosing brown rice flour.

Directions:

1. Preheat oven to 350°F.

2. Cut the sweet potatoes into 2 to 3 inch pieces. Steam the sweet potatoes until they are soft (about 10 minutes). Then, puree or mash them, adding 2 to 4 tablespoons of water if needed to make smooth.

3. Mix together the dry ingredients (cornmeal, flour, baking powder, baking soda, and salt) in a bowl.

4. In a separate bowl mix together the sweet potato puree, egg, maple syrup and melted coconut oil or butter.

5. Add the dry ingredients to the wet ingredients and gently mix. Batter should be thick and moist.

6. Grease a 9″ x 13″ pan and pour batter into pan. Bake for 25 to 30 minutes or until an inserted knife comes out clean.

Tips:

*   If you are avoiding eggs, consider the following egg substitutions for baking:

    1 egg = ¼ cup unsweetened applesauce = 1 tablespoon ground flaxseed with ¼ cup hot water; let sit for 5 minutes to create a gelatinous consistency.

Delicata Squash Over Broccoli and Quinoa

Enjoy this simple, yet savory dish in the fall and winter when delicata squash is generally in season. Delicata squash is oblong and yellow colored with distinct bright green stripes. It is considered the delicata, or delicate squash, because its outer skin is easier to cut through. The skin can even be eaten, unlike most of its squash relatives. Also, it doesn't take quite as long to cook. If you are new to eating squash, the delicata is a great introduction to this vitamin-rich food. Yet, any variety of squash (see **Baked Acorn Squash**) pairs well with broccoli and quinoa, along with this tasty dressing.

3 cups water

1½ cup quinoa

3 to 4 delicata squash

¼ cup coconut oil

1 medium onion, diced

3 cloves garlic, peeled and minced

6 cups chopped broccoli florets

¼ cup sunflower seeds

¾ teaspoon salt

½ teaspoon black pepper

Directions:

1. To prepare the quinoa: Bring 3 cups of water to a boil in a medium saucepan. Add 1 ½ cups quinoa and return to a boil. Reduce heat to simmer, cover, and cook for 12 to 15 minutes, until water is absorbed. Remove from heat. Let the quinoa sit for five minutes and then fluff with a fork.

2. Mix dressing ingredients together in a bowl and whisk.

3. Cut the delicata squash lengthwise, remove seeds with a spoon, and cut squash into 1-inch cubes with the skin on.

4. Heat 2 tablespoons of oil in a pan on low-medium heat. Add squash to pan and cook until soft, approximately 10 minutes.

5. Heat a separate pan over medium heat and add 2 tablespoons of oil. Sauté the onions until translucent, about 3 to 5 minutes.

6. Add the garlic and broccoli florets. Sauté for another 5 minutes until broccoli is softened, yet still brightly colored. Add a small amount of the dressing to help steam the broccoli. Add sunflower seeds in the last few minutes. Add salt and pepper to taste.

7. Create a healthy FAME Plate: serve 1 to 2 cups of broccoli on top of ½ cup quinoa. Add ½ to 1 cup of cooked squash. Drizzle dressing over plate.

DRESSING INGREDIENTS:

½ cup extra virgin olive oil

¼ cup balsalmic vinegar

1 teaspoon maple syrup

1 teaspoon dijon mustard

2 teaspoons dried herbs (sage, thyme or rosemary)

¼ teaspoon salt

⅛ teaspoon black pepper

Servings: 4 to 6

Tips:

- Oven alternative: Spread 1-inch cubes of delicate squash onto a baking sheet or baking pan and coat with melted coconut oil, salt, and pepper. Then bake at 350°F for 20 to 30 minutes until softened.

- Save your squash seeds. Remove squash strings, rinse the seeds and pat them dry. Coat in a small amount of coconut oil or extra virgin olive oil, salt, and add your favorite spices. Bake at 275°F for approximately 15 minutes or until seeds are crisp. Sprinkle on top of this meal, or save for a tasty snack.

Baked Acorn Squash

Acorn squash, a dark green squash in the shape of an acorn, is a delicious alternative to the delicata squash, although it requires a different preparation. The acorn squash is best prepared baked in the oven. This squash tends to be seasonal in the fall and winter, which is the perfect time to enjoy this sweet vegetable because of its immune-supporting nutrients. Squash provides a good source of beta-carotene, a precursor to vitamin A, which supports a healthy immune system. Its skin is tougher than a delicata squash, so the cooked squash is often removed from the skin to eat.

Directions:

1. Preheat the oven to 350°F.

2. Carefully cut acorn squash in half with a sharp knife and remove inner seeds.

3. Rub the open face of each squash with a mixture of 1 teaspoon of coconut oil or melted butter mixed with 1 teaspoon of maple syrup.

4. Cut a flat edge on the underside of the squash to keep it upright and even. Place squash into a baking dish. Add a pinch of salt to the face of the squash.

5. Prior to putting the baking dish in the oven, add water to cover the bottom of the dish to a depth of approximately ¼ inch.

6. Bake for approximately 45 minutes. Check on squash every 10 to 15 minutes and add water if needed. When fully cooked, scoop out the squash with a spoon for serving.

i n g r e d i e n t s

2 acorn squash
2 teaspoons melted coconut oil or
*   melted butter*
2 teaspoons maple syrup
salt, a pinch

Servings: 4 to 6

ingredients

4 cups water

2 cup brown rice

2 tablespoons coconut oil

1 yellow onion, chopped

4 cloves garlic, peeled and minced

2 tablespoons peeled and minced
    ginger

1 tablespoon cumin

2 tablespoons curry powder

¼ teaspoon ground cardamom

1 jalapeno pepper, finely chopped
    (optional)

2 cups red lentils

8 cups low-sodium vegetable broth

1½ cups diced tomatoes (fresh or
    canned)

5 cups finely chopped spinach leaves

1 teaspoon salt

½ cup chopped fresh cilantro

Servings: 8 to 10

Spiced Red Lentils (Dal) with Spinach

Dal is a traditional Indian dish, commonly made with lentils. Nothing compares to this warming, spicy dish on a cool fall or winter day. Cardamom is an amazing and powerful spice that is also used in chai tea. Cardamom can be expensive, but a small amount can be purchased in the bulk spice section at the grocery store. Curry powder is a spice mixture that contains turmeric, which gives it a bright yellow-colored base. Turmeric contains curcumin, a very potent anti-inflammatory. Be creative and add other vegetables to this Dal such as sweet potato, cauliflower, or green peas. The addition of finely chopped dark green leafy greens complements this delicious Dal.

Directions:

1. Place water and rice into a pot and bring to a boil. Reduce heat to simmer and allow rice to cook for 35 to 40 minutes until water is absorbed. Remove from heat and fluff with a fork.

2. Heat a large pot over medium heat and add oil. Add onions and sauté until translucent, about 3 to 5 minutes.

3. Add garlic, ginger, cumin, curry powder, cardamom, and jalapeno (optional) to the onions, stirring often, until fragrant, about 2 minutes.

4. Add lentils, 6 cups of broth, and diced tomatoes to the pot and bring to a boil. Reduce heat to medium-low. Cover and simmer, stirring often, until lentils are soft (about 15 to 20 minutes). Add spinach and salt during the last 3 minutes of cooking. Add more broth, if needed, for desired consistency.

5. Serve dal over brown rice. Add chopped cilantro over dal.

Tips:

- If you substitute green lentils, they take longer to cook—around 30 to 40 minutes. If adding other ingredients—sweet potato, peas, cauliflower, add them with the lentils and broth.

Black Bean Caribbean Pumpkin Soup

Many of us feel inspired to include pumpkin in our meals during the fall months. This creamy soup brings together pumpkin, coconut, and black beans with all the right spices to create a very satisfying flavor. While canned pumpkin will suffice in this soup, consider baking a pumpkin and creating homemade pumpkin puree. Be sure to use a *pie* or *baking* pumpkin for this recipe; the traditional Halloween pumpkins won't be very tasty.

Directions:

1. Carefully slice the pumpkin in half, scoop out seeds, and chop pumpkin into large chunks. Steam the pumpkin chunks until soft, about 10 minutes. Let pumpkin cool, remove the skin, and puree in a food processor or a blender until smooth.

2. Heat a large pot over medium heat and add oil. Sauté onions until translucent, about 3 to 5 minutes.

3. Add garlic, cumin, salt, cayenne, and cinnamon and stir for 2 minutes.

4. Add the black beans, pumpkin, tomatoes, coconut milk and broth into the pot. Simmer for 10 minutes allowing flavors to combine and ingredients to soften.

5. If you prefer a smooth soup, use an immersion blender in the pot or pour soup into a blender and blend to desired consistency.

6. Garnish with cilantro, roasted pumpkin seeds, and avocado.

Tips:

- If you are using canned pumpkin puree, coconut milk, or diced tomato, look for these items in glass jars or in cans or packaging that are BPA-free.

- To boost the protein in this soup, add ½ pound of cooked ground turkey or chicken to the final soup.

ingredients

2 cups pureed pumpkin

1 tablespoon coconut oil or butter

1 yellow onion, chopped

2 cloves garlic, peeled and minced

1 tablespoon cumin

1 teaspoon salt

½ teaspoon cayenne (optional)

½ teaspoon cinnamon

3 cups cooked or canned black beans

2 large tomatoes, diced or 1 can (14.5 ounces) diced tomatoes

1 cup full-fat canned coconut milk

3 cups low-sodium vegetable broth

¼ cup chopped fresh cilantro

Pumpkin seeds, sliced avocado, or sour cream (optional toppings)

Servings: 6 to 8

ingredients

- To cook the pumpkin seeds for a topping, preheat oven to 275°F. Clean the seeds, and pat them dry. Coat them in a small amount of oil and salt, and then spread them evenly on a baking sheet. Bake for 15 to 20 minutes until crispy.

Nutrition Facts:

- Pumpkin pulp is a rich source of magnesium and vitamins (B's and C). Pumpkin seeds are a rich source of immune-boosting zinc, as well as tryptophan, the precursor to the *feel good* neurotransmitter, serotonin.

Roasted Brussels Sprouts

4 cups quartered Brussels sprouts
¼ cup refined coconut oil, melted
1 cup pecans
4 cloves garlic, peeled and minced
¼ teaspoon salt
¼ teaspoon cinnamon
¼ teaspoon cumin
¼ teaspoon cayenne pepper (optional)

Servings: 4

This simple recipe can win over any Brussels sprouts doubter.

Directions:

1. Preheat oven to 400°F.
2. Chop Brussels sprouts into quarters and place in a bowl.
3. Massage or stir melted coconut oil into Brussels sprouts. Add pecans, garlic, salt, cumin, cinnamon, and cayenne (optional) to the Brussels sprouts and stir.
4. Spread ingredients onto baking pan. Cover with aluminum foil.
5. Place in oven and bake for 30 minutes. Remove aluminum foil and turn sprouts with a spatula. Return to the oven for an additional 10 to 15 minutes, or until Brussels sprouts are soft (check with a fork).

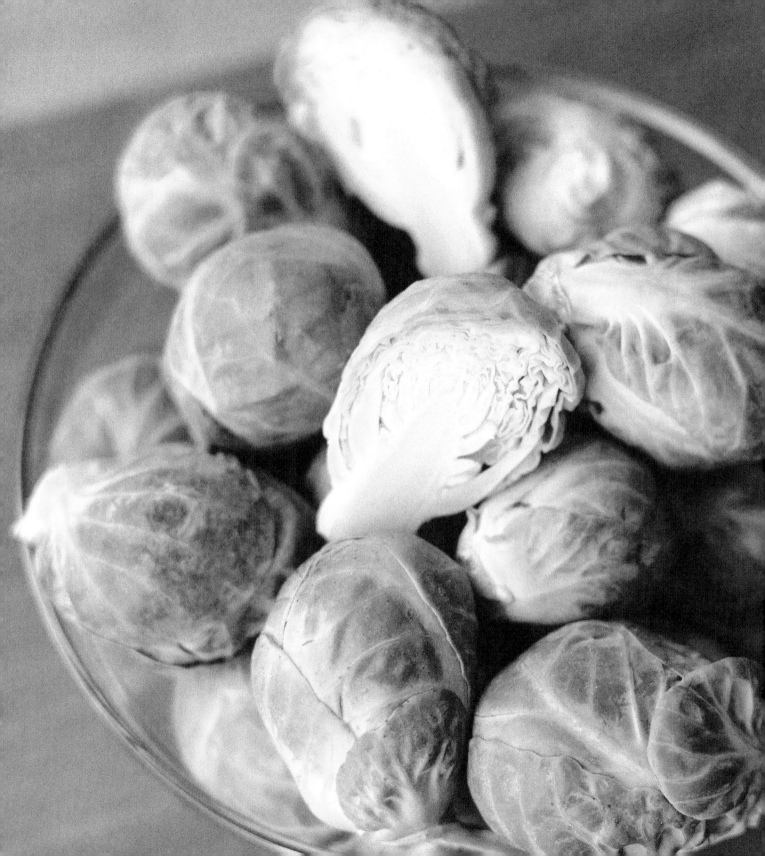

References

Preface

1. Barnes PM, Bloom B, Nahin R. "Complementary and alternative medicine use among adults and children: United States, 2007." *CDC National Health Statistics Report #12.* December 10, 2008.

2. Stone, Mike. "What patients want from their doctors." *BMJ.* 2003 June 14; 326(7402): 1294.

3. Adams K, Lindell K, Kohlmeier M, Zeisel S. "Status of nutrition education in medical schools". *Am J Clin Nutr.* 2006 April; 83(4): 941S-944S.

Introduction

1. Johnston B, Kanters S, Bandayrel K, Wu P, Naji F, Siemieniuk R et al. "Comparison of weight loss among named diet programs in over-weight and obese adults, a meta-analysis." *JAMA.* 2014; 312(9):923-933.

2. Pawlak R, Lester SE, Babatunde T. "The prevalence of cobalamin deficiency among vegetarians assessed by serum vitamin B12: a review of literature." *Eur J Clin Nutr.* 2014 May; 68(5):541-8.

3. McCarron et al. "Community-based priorities for improving nutrition and physical activity in childhood." *Pediatrics.* 2010 Nov 1; 126 (2): S73-S89.

4. Larson NI, Neumark-Sztainer D, Hannan PJ, Story M. "Family meals during adolescence are associated with higher diet quality and healthful meal patterns during young adulthood." *J Am Diet Assoc.* 2007 Sep; 107(9):1502-10.

5. Larson NI, Nelson MC, Neumark-Sztainer D, Story M, Hannan PJ. "Making time for meals: meal structure and associations with dietary intake in young adults." *J Am Diet Assoc.* 2009 Jan; 109(1):72-9.

Chapter 1: The Wisdom Of Traditional Diets

1. "The problem of noncommunicable diseases and CDC's role in combating them". *CDC.* n.d. Retrieved 16 Sept 2014.

2. "10 facts on non-communicable disease." *World Health Organization.* n.d. Retrieved 16 Sept 2014.

3. Mercader J. "Mozambican grass seed consumption during the middle stone age." *Science.* 2009 Dec 18;326(5960):1680-3.

4. Hotz C, Gibson R. "Traditional food-processing and preparation practices to enhance the bioavailability of micronutrients in plant-based diets". *J. Nutr.* April 2007; vol. 137 no. 4 1097-1100.

5. American Association For The Advancement Of Science. "Diet and disease in cattle: high-grain feed may promote illness and harmful bacteria." *Science Daily.* 11 May 2001.

6. Luciano G, Moloney AP, Priolo A, Röhrle FT, Vasta V, Biondi L, López-Andrés P, Grasso S, Monahan FJ. "Vitamin E and polyunsaturated fatty acids in bovine muscle and the oxidative stability of beef from cattle receiving grass or concentrate-based rations. " *J Anim Sci.* 2011 Nov;89(11):3759-68.

7. Daley C, Abbot A, Doyle P, Nader G, Larson S. "A review of fatty acid profiles and antioxidant content in grass-fed and grain-fed beef." *Nutr J.* 2010 Mar 10; 9:10.

8. He ML et al. "Feeding flaxseed in grass hay and barley silage diets to beef cows increases alpha-linolenic acid and its biohydrogenation intermediates in subcutaneous fat." *J Anim Sci*. 2012 Feb;90(2):592-604. doi: 10.2527/jas.2011-4281.

9. Westin Price. Excerpt from Prologue from *Nutrition and Physical Degeneration*, 8th Edition. Price-Pottenger Nutrition Foundation, 2008.

Chapter 2: Nourish Yourself With Fat

1. Grootveld M, Silwood C, Addis P, Claxson A, Serra B, Viana M. "Health effects of oxidized heated oils." *Foodservice Research International*. 2001; (13): 41–55.

2. Jakobsen MU, O'Reilly EJ, Heitmann BL, et al. "Major types of dietary fat and risk of coronary heart disease: a pooled analysis of 11 cohort studies." *Am J Clin Nutr*. 2009;89:1425-1432.

3. Grimm MO, Rothhaar TL, Grösgen S, Burg VK, Hundsdörfer B, Haupenthal VJ, Friess P, Kins S, Grimm HS, Hartmann T. "Trans fatty acids enhance amyloidogenic processing of the Alzheimer amyloid precursor protein (APP)." *J Nutr Biochem*. 2012 Oct; 23(10):1214-23.

4. Wang Q, Imamura F, Lemaitre RN, Rimm EB, Wang M, King IB, Song X, Siscovick D, Mozaffarian D. "Plasma phospholipid trans-fatty acids levels, cardiovascular diseases, and total mortality: the cardiovascular health study." *J Am Heart Assoc*. 2014 Aug 27;3(4).

5. "Letter report on dietary reference intakes for trans fatty acids: drawn from the report on dietary reference intakes for energy, carbohydrate, fiber, fat, fatty acids, cholesterol, protein, and amino acids. A report of the panel of macronutrients, subcommittees on upper reference levels of nutrients and on interpretation and uses of dietary reference intakes, and the standing committee on the scientific evaluation of dietary reference intakes." Food and Nutrition Board. Institute of Medicine. Copyright 2002 by National Academy of Sciences.

6. Forouhi NG, Koulman A, Sharp SJ, et al. "Differences in the prospective association between individual plasma phospholipid saturated fatty acids and incident type 2 diabetes: the EPIC-InterAct case-cohort study." *Lancet Diabetes Endocrinol*. 2014;2:810-818.

7. Scirica B, Cannon C. "Treatment of Elevated Cholesterol". *Circulation*. 2005; 111: e360-e363.

8. Sachdeva A, Cannon C, Deedwania P, LaBresh K, Smith S, Dai D, Hernandez A, Fonarow G. "Lipid levels in patients hospitalized with coronary artery disease: An analysis of 136,905 hospitalizations in Get With The Guidelines". *American Heart Journal*. 2009 January; Volume 157, Issue 1, Pages 111-117.e2.

9. Tedders SH, Fokong KD, McKenzie LE, Wesley C, Yu L, Zhang J. "Low cholesterol is associated with depression among US household population." *J Affect Disord*. 2011 Dec; 135(1-3):115-21.

10. Fernandez ML. "Effects of eggs on plasma lipoproteins in healthy populations." *Food Funct*. 2010 Nov;1(2):156-60.

11. Jones, PJ. "Dietary cholesterol and the risk of cardiovascular disease in patients: a review of the Harvard Egg Study and other data." *International Journal of Clinical Practice*. 2009 October; Vol 63, Issue Supplement s163, pp. 1-8.

12. Kiecolt-Glaser JK, Belury MA, Porter K, Beversdorf DQ, Lemeshow S, Glaser R. "Depressive symptoms, omega-6:omega-3 fatty acids, and inflammation in older adults." *Psychosom Med*. 2007 Apr;69(3):217-24. Epub 2007 Mar 30.

13. Naito Y, Nagata T, Takano Y, et al. "Rapeseed oil ingestion and exacerbation of hypertension-related conditions in stroke prone spontaneously hypertensive rats." *Toxicology*. 2003 May 3; 187(2-3):205-16.

14. Przybylski O, Aladedunye FA. "Formation of trans fats during food preparation" *Can J Diet Pract Res*. 2012; 73(2): 98-101.

15. Papamandjaris AA, MacDougall DE, Jones PJ. "Medium chain fatty acid metabolism and energy expenditure: obesity treatment implications." *Life Sci.* 1998;62(14):1203-15.

16. Bazzano L, Hu T, Reynolds K, Yao L, Bunol C, Liu Y, et al. "Effects of low-carbohydrate and low-fat diets: A randomized trial." *Ann Intern Med.* 2014;161(5):309-318.

17. German and Dillard. "Saturated fats: what dietary intake?" *AM J Clin Nutr.* 2004; 80:550-9.

Chapter 3: Nourish Yourself With Carbohydrates

1. Leach, JD. "Evolutionary perspective on dietary intake of fiber and colorectal cancer." *Eur. J. Clin. Nutr.* 2007; 61: 140-142.

2. Brown L, Rosner B, Willet W, Sacks F. "Cholesterol-lowering effects of dietary fiber: a meta-analysis." *The American Journal of Clinical Nutrition.* 1999; Vol 69 no 1, pp 30-42.

3. Bazzano LA. "Effects of soluble dietary fiber on low-density lipoprotein cholesterol and coronary heart disease risk." *Curr Atheroscler Rep.* 2008 Dec;10(6): pp. 473-7.

4. Cho SS, Qi L, Rahey GC, Klurfeld DM. "Consumption of cereal fiber, mixtures of whole grains and bran, and whole grains and risk reduction in type 2 diabetes, obesity, and cardiovascular disease." *Am J Clin Nutr.* 2013 Aug; 98(2): 594-619.

5. Fung TT, Hu FB, Pereira MA, et al. "Whole–grain intake and the risk of Type II diabetes: a prospective study in men." *Am J Clin Nutr.* 2002; 76:535–40.

6. Liu S, Willett WC, Stampfer MJ, et al. "A prospective study of dietary glycemic load, carbohydrate intake, and risk of coronary heart disease in US women." *Am J Clin Nutr.* 2000; 71:1455–61.

7. Schulze MB, Liu S, Rimm EB, Manson JE, Willett WC, Hu FB. "Glycemic index, glycemic load, and dietary fiber intake and incidence of Type II diabetes in younger and middle-aged women." *Am J Clin Nutr.* 2004; 80:348–56.

8. Kimm SY. "The role of dietary fiber in the development and treatment of childhood obesity." *Pediatrics.* 1995;96 (5 Pt 2):1010–4.

9. Rezazadeh A, Rashidkhani B. "The association of general and central obesity with major dietary patterns in adult women living in Tehran, Iran." *ARYA Atheroscler.* 2010 Spring; 6(1): 23–30.

10. "Dietary, functional, and total fiber. Dietary reference intakes for energy, carbohydrates, fiber, fat, fatty acids, cholesterol, protein, and amino acids." Institute of Medicine. 2002; 265-334.

Chapter 5: Reading Food Labels

1. Mozaffarian D, Abdollahi M, Campos H, Houshiarrad A, Willet WC. "Consumption of trans fats and estimated effects on coronary heart disease in Iran." *Eur J Clin Nutr.* 2007 Aug; 61(8):1004-10.

2. Bowman GL, Silbert LC, HOwieson D, Dodge HH, Traver MG, Frei B, Kaye JA, Shannon J, Quinn JF. "Nutrient biomarker patterns, cognitive function, and MRI measures of brain aging." *Neurology.* 2012 Jan 24;78(4):241-9.

3. "Food additives". Asthma and Allergy Foundation of America. n.d. Retrieved September 18, 2014.

4. Bateman B. "The effects of a double blind, placebo controlled, artificial food colorings and benzoate preservative challenge on hyperactivity in a general population sample of preschool children." *Arch Dis Child.* 2004 Jun;89(6):506-11.

5. Stevens LJ, Kuczek T, Burgess J, Stochelski M, Arnold LE, Galland L. "Mechanisms of behavioral, atopic, and other reactions to artificial food colors in children." *Nutr Rev.* 2013 May; 71(5):268-81.

6. Stevens LJ, Kuczek T, Burgess JR, Hurt E, Arnold LE. "Dietary sensitivities and ADHD symptoms: thirty-five years of research." *Clin Pediatr* (Phila). 2011 Apr; 50(4):279-93.

7. Olney JW. "Excitotoxins in foods." *Neurotoxicology.* 1994 Fall; 15(3):535-44.

8. Alderman MH, Cohen HW. "Dietary sodium intake and cardiovascular mortality: controversy resolved?" *Curr Hypertens Rep.* 2012 Jun;14(3):193-201.

9. Chobanian AV, Hill M. "National heart, lung, and blood institute workshop on sodium and blood pressure : a critical review of current scientific evidence." *Hypertension.* 2000;35(4):858-863.

10. Food and Nutrition Board, Institute of Medicine. "Sodium and chloride. Dietary reference intakes for water, potassium, sodium, chloride, and sulfate." Washington, D.C.: National Academies Press; 2005:269-423.

11. Anna Vallverdu-Queralt, Jauregui O, Medina-Remon A, Lamuela-Raventos RM. "Evaluation of a method to characterize the phenolic profile of organic and conventional tomatoes." *Journal of Agricultural and Food Chemistry*, 2013; 60 (13): 3373.

12. Daley C, Abbott A, Doyle P, Nader G, and Larson S. "A review of fatty acid profiles and antioxidant content in grass-fed and grain-fed beef." *Nutr J.* 2010; 9: 10.

13. "US sour on EU biofood vote". CBS News, 25 June 2003. Retrieved September 22, 2014.

14. Nordlee, J.A, Taylor S, Townsend J, Thomas L, Bush R. "Identification of a brazil-nut allergen in transgenic soybeans." *The New England Journal of Medicine*, 334 (11): 688-692.

15. "Biological confinement of genetically engineered organisms". National Academy Press, 2004.

16. Bhan A, Hussain I, Ansari KI, Bobzean SA, Perrotti LI, Mandal SS. "Bisphenol-A and diethylstilbestrol exposure induces the expression of breast cancer associated long noncoding RNA HOTAIR in vitro and in vivo." *J Steroid Biochem Mol Biol.* 2014 May;141:160-70.

17. Tarapore P, Ying J, Ouyang B, Burke B, Bracken B, Ho SM. "Exposure to bisphenol A correlates with early-onset prostate cancer and promotes centrosome amplification and anchorage-independent growth in vitro." *PLoS One.* 2014 Mar 3;9(3):e90332.

Chapter 6: The FAME Plate

1. Ello-Martin JA, Ledikwe J, Rolls B. "The influence of food portion size and energy density on energy intake: implications for weight management." *Am J Clin Nutr.* 2005 Jul;82(1 Suppl):236S-241S.

2. Ello-Martin JA, Ledikwe J, Rolls B. "The influence of food portion size and energy density on energy intake: implications for weight management." *Am J Clin Nutr.* 2005 Jul;82(1 Suppl):236S-241S.

3. Smit LA, Baylin A, Campos H. "Conjugated linoleic acid in adipose tissue and risk of myocardial infaction." *Am J Clin Nutr.* 2010 Jul: 92 (1): 34-40.

4. Hebeisen DF, Hoeflin F, Reusch HP, Junker E, Lauterburg BH. "Increased concentrations of omega-3 fatty acids in milk and platelet rich plasma of grass-fed cows." *Int J Vitam Nutr Res.* 1993;63(3):229-33.

5.   CA Daley, Abbott A, Doyle PA, Nader GA, Larson A. "A review of fatty acid profiles and antioxidant content in grass-fed and grain-fed beef." *Nutr J.* 2010 Mar 10; 9:10.

6.   Feskanich D, Willet WC, Stampfer MJ, Colditz GA. "Milk, dietary calcium, and bone fractures in women: a 12-year prospective study." *Am J Public Health.* 1997;87:992-7.

7.   Genkinger JM, Hunter DJ, Spiegelman D, Anderson KE, Arslan A, Beeson WL, Buring JE, et al. "Dairy products and ovarian cancer: a pooled analysis of 12 cohort studies." *Cancer Epidemiol Biomarkers Prev.* 2006; 15:364–72.

8.   World Cancer Research Fund, American Institute for Cancer Research. "Food, nutrition, physical activity, and the prevention of cancer: a global perspective." Washington DC: AICR, 2007.

9.   Giovannucci E, Rimm EB, Wolk A, et al. "Calcium and fructose intake in relation to risk of prostate cancer." *Cancer Res.* 1998; 58:442–447.

10. Giovannucci E, Liu Y, Platz EA, Stampfer MJ, Willett WC. "Risk factors for prostate cancer incidence and progression in the Health Professionals Follow-up Study." *International Journal of Cancer.* 2007; 121:1571–78.

11. Heaney RP, Weaver CM. "Calcium absorption from kale." *Am J Clin Nutr.* 1990;51:656-657.

12. Weaver CM, Plawecki KL. "Dietary calcium: adequacy of a vegetarian diet." *Am J Clin Nutr.* 1994; 59(suppl):1238S-41S.

13. Ebbeling C, Swain J, Feldman H, Wond W, Hachey D, Garcia-Lago E, Ludwig D. "Effects of dietary composition on energy expenditure during weight loss maintenance". *JAMA.* 2012; 307, No. 24: 2627-2634.

Chapter 7: Strategies For Healthy Digestion

1.   O'Keefe JH, Gheewala NM, O'Keefe JO. "Dietary strategies for improving post-prandial glucose, lipids, inflammation, and cardiovascular health." *J Am Coll Cardiol.* 2008;51 (3): 249-255.

2.   Savage DC. "Microbial ecology of the gastrointenstinal tract". *Annual Review of Microbiology.* 1977; 31:107-133.

3.   Gill SR, Pop M, DeBoy RT, Eckburg PB, Turnbaugh PJ, Samuel BS, et al. "Metagenomic analysis of the human distal gut microbiome." *Science.* 2006; 312: 1357.

4.   Hill MJ. "Intestinal flora and endogenous vitamin synthesis". *European Journal of Cancer Prevention.* 1977; 6 (Suppl. 1): S43.

5.   Leahy SC, Higgins DG, Fitzgerald GF, van Sinderen D. "Getting better with bifidobacteria". *Journal of Applied Microbiology.* 2005; 98: 1303.

6.   Hopper LV, Wong MH, Thelin A, Hansson L, Falk PG, Gordon JI. "Molecular analysis of commensal host-microbial relationships in the intestine". *Science.* 2001; 291: 881.

7.   Kelly D, Conway S, Aminov R. "Commensal gut bacteria: mechanism of immune modulation". *Trends in Immunology.* 2005; 26: 326.

8.   Reid G, Jass J, Subulsky T, McCormick J. "Potential uses of probiotics in clinical oractice". *Clin Microbiol Rev.* Oct 2003; 16(4): 658–672.

Chapter 8: Balancing Blood Sugar

1. Rimm EB, Klatsky A, Grobbee D, Stampfer MJ. "Review of moderate alcohol consumption and reduced risk of coronary heart disease: is the effect due to beer, wine, or spirits." *BMJ*. 1996 Mar 23;312(7033):731-6.

2. Metcalf PA, Scragg RK, Jackson R. "Light to moderate alcohol consumption is protective for type 2 diabetes mellitus in normal weight and overweight individuals but not the obese." *J Obes*. 2014; 2014: 634587.

3. Lando L.J. Koppes, , Jacqueline M. Dekker, Henk F.J. Hendriks, Lex M. Bouter, and Robert J. Heine. "Moderate alcohol consumption lowers the risk of type 2 diabetes: A meta-analysis of prospective observational studies." *Diabetes Care*. March 2005; 28(3): 719-725.

4. Vasanthi HR, Parameswari RP, DeLeiris J, Das DK. "Health benefits of wine and alcohol from neuroprotection to heart health." *Front Biosci* (Elite Ed). 2012 Jan 1;4:1505-12.

5. De Oliveira E Silva ER, Foster D, McGee Harper M, Seidman CE, Smith JD, Breslow JL, Brinton EA. "Alcohol consumption raises HDL cholesterol levels by increasing the transport rate of apolipoproteins A-I and A-II." *Circulation*. 2000 Nov 7;102(19):2347-52.

6. Avogaro A, Fontana P, Valerio A, et al. "Alcohol impairs insulin sensitivity in normal subjects." *Diabetes Res*. 1987; 5: 23–7.

7. Goude D, Fagerberg B, Hulthe J. "Alcohol consumption, the metabolic syndrome and insulin resistance in 58-year-old clinically healthy men (AIR Study)." *Clin Sci* (Lond). 2002; 102: 345–52.

8. Flanagan D, Moore V, Godsland I, Cockington R, Robinson J, Phillips D. "Alcohol consumption and insulin resistance in young adults." *Eur J Clin Invest*. 2000; 30: 297–301.

9. Franke A, Nakchbandi IA, Schneider A, Harder H, Singer MV. "The effect of ethanol and alcoholic beverages on gastric emptying of solid meals in humans." *Alcohol Alcohol*. 2005 May-Jun;40(3):187-93.

10. Roswall N, Weiderpass E. "Alcohol as a risk factor for cancer: existing evidence in a global perspective." *J Prev Med Public Health*. 2015 Jan;48(1):1-9.

11. Esteghamati A, Aryan Z, Esteghamati A, Nakhjavani M. "Differences in vitamin D concentration between metabolically healthy and un-healthy obese adults: Associations with inflammatory and cardiometabolic markers in 4391 subjects." *Diabetes Metab*. 2014 May 5. pii: S1262-3636(14)00046-9.

12. Anderson RA. "Chromium, glucose intolerance and diabetes." *J Am Coll Nutr*. 1998 Dec;17(6):548-55.

Chapter 9: Exploring Sweeteners

1. "Dietary quality of American school-age children by school lunch participation status: data from the National Health and Nutrition Examination Survey, 1999-2004." USDA Food and Nutrition Services. n.d. Retrieved July 2008.

2. "Consumption of sugar drinks in the United States, 2005–2008". *CDC and Prevention*. NCHS Data Brief. Retrieved August 2011.

3. Lecoultre V, Egli L, Carrel G, Theytaz F, Kreis R, Schneiter P, et al. "Effects of fructose and glucose overfeeding on hepatic insulin sensitivity and intrahepatic lipids in healthy humans." *Obesity* (Silver Spring). 2013 Apr;21(4):782-5.

4. Borjian A, Ferrari CC, Anouf A, Touyz L. "Pop-cola acids and tooth erosion: an in vitro, in vivo, electron-microscopic, and clinical report." *Int J Dent*. 2010; 2010:957842.

5. Tucker KL, Morita K, Qiao N, Hannan MT, Cupples LA, Kiel DP. "Colas, but not other carbonated beverages, are associated with low bone mineral density in older women: The Framingham Osteoporosis Study." *Am J Clin Nutr.* 2006 Oct;84(4):936-42.

6. Mahmood M, Saleh A, Al-Alawi F, Ahmed F. "Health effects of soda drinking in adolescent girls in the United Arab Emirates." *J Crit Care.* 2008 Sep;23(3):434-40.

7. Schultze MB, Manson JE, Ludwig DS, Colditz GA, Stampfer MJ, Willet WC, Hu FB. " Sugar-sweetened beverages, weight gain, and incidence of Type II diabetes in young and middle-aged women." *JAMA.* 2004 Aug 25; 292(8):927-34.

8. Lecoultre V, Egli L, Carrel G, Theytaz F, Kreis R, Schneiter P, et al. "Effects of fructose and glucose overfeeding on hepatic insulin sensitivity and intrahepatic lipids in healthy humans." *Obesity* (Silver Spring). 2013 Apr;21(4):782-5.

9. Lustig RH. "Fructose: It's "Alcohol without the buzz". *Adv Nutr.* 2013 Mar 1;4(2):226-35.

10. Tappy L, Le KA, Tran C, Paquot N. "Fructose and metabolic diseases: new findings, new questions." *Nutrition.* 2010 Nov-Dec;26(11-12):1044-9.

11. B. Anton SD, Martin CK, Han H, Coulon S, Cefalu WT, Geiselman P, Williamson DA. "Effects of stevia, aspartame, and sucrose on food intake, satiety, and postprandial glucose and insulin levels." *Appetite.* 2010 Aug;55(1):37-43.

12. Nettleton JA, Lutsey PL, Wang Y, Lima JA, Michos ED, Jacobs DR Jr. "Diet soda intake and risk of incident metabolic syndrome and type 2 diabetes in the multi-ethnic study of atherosclerosis (MESA)." *Diabetes Care.* 2009 April 32 (4): 688-694.

13. "Artificial sweeteners and cancer". National Cancer Institute at the National Institute of Health, 5 August 2009. Web. 22 September 2014.

14. "Artificial sweeteners and cancer". National Cancer Institute at the National Institute of Health, 5 August 2009. Web. 22 September 2014.

15. Pepino MY, Tiemann CD, Patterson BW, Wice BM, Klein S. "Sucralose affects glycemic and hormonal responses to an oral glucose load." *Diabetes Care.* 2013 Sept; 36(9):2530-5.

16. Nettleton JA, Lutsey PL, Wang Y, Lima JA, Michos ED, Jacobs DR Jr. "Diet soda intake and risk of incident metabolic syndrome and type 2 diabetes in the multi-ethnic study of atherosclerosis (MESA)." *Diabetes Care.* 2009 April 32 (4): 688-694.

17. Sakurai M, Nakamura K, Miura K, Takamura T, Yoshita K, Nagasawa SY. "Sugar-sweetened beverage and diet soda consumption and the 7-year risk for Type II diabetes mellitus in middle-aged Japanese men." *Eur J Nutr.* 2014 Feb;53(1):251-8.

18. Fowler SP, Williams K, Resendez RG, Hunt KJ, Hazuda HP, Stern MP. "Fueling the obesity epidemic? Artificially sweetened beverage use and long-term weight gain." *Obesity* (Silver Spring, Md.) 2008;16:1894–1900.

19. Liem DG, de Graaf C. "Sweet and sour preferences in young children and adults: role of repeated exposure." *Physiol Behav.* 2004;83:421–429.

20. Mennella JA, Jagnow CP, Beauchamp GK. "Prenatal and postnatal flavor learning by human infants." *Pediatrics.* 2001 Jun;107(6):E88.

Chapter 10: Benefits Of Breakfast

1. Dalkara T, Kiliç K. "How does fasting trigger migraine? A hypothesis." *Curr Pain Headache Rep.* 2013 Oct;17 (10): 368.

2. Fuse Y, Hirao A, Kuroda H, Otsuka M, Tahara Y, Shibata S. "Differential roles of breakfast only (one meal per day) and a bigger breakfast with a small dinner (two meals per day) in mice fed a high-fat diet with regard to induced obesity and lipid metabolism." *Journal of Circadian Rhythms*. 2012; May 15;10(1):4.

3. Wyatt HR, Grunwald GK, Mosca CL, Klem ML, Wing RR, Hill JO. "Long-term weight loss and breakfast in subjects in the National Weight Control Registry." *Obes Res*. 2002 Feb;10(2):78-82.

4. Chaplin K, Smith A. "Breakfast and snacks: associations with cognitive failures, minor injuries, accidents and stress." *Nutrients*. 2011 May;3(5):515-28.

5. Cahill LE, Chiuve SE, Mekary RA, Jensen MK, Flint AJ, Hu FB, Rimm EB. "Prospective study of breakfast eating and incident coronary heart disease in a cohort of male US health professionals." *Circulation*. 2013 Jul 23;128(4):337-43.

6. Mekary RA, Giovannucci E, Cahill L, Willett WC, van Dam RM, Hu FB. "Eating patterns and type 2 diabetes risk in older women: breakfast consumption and eating frequency." *Am J Clin Nutr*. 2013 Aug;98(2):436-43.

7. de la Hunty A, Gibson S, Ashwell M. "Does regular breakfast cereal consumption help children and adolescents stay slimmer? A systematic review and meta-analysis." *Obes Facts* 2013:6 (1) 70-85.

8. Lustig, Robert H. "Fat Chance. Beating the odds against sugar, processed food, obesity, and disease." 2012; Hudson Street Press, pp142-143.

9. Deshmukh-Taskar PR, Nicklas TA, O'Neil CE, Keast DR, Radcliffe JD, Cho S. "The relationship of breakfast skipping and type of breakfast consumption with nutrient intake and weight status in children and adolescents: the National Health and Nutrition Examination Survey 1999-2006." *J Am Diet Assoc*. 2010 June; 110 (6): 869-78.

10. Sjöberg A, Hallberg L, Höglund D, Hulthén L. "Meal pattern, food choice, nutrient intake and lifestyle factors in The Göteborg Adolescence Study." *Eur J Clin Nutr*. 2003 Dec;57(12):1569-78.

11. Widenhorn-Müller K, Hille K, Klenk J, Weiland U. "Influence of having breakfast on cognitive performance and mood in 13-20 year-old high school students: results of a crossover trial." *Pediatrics*. 2008 Aug; 122 (2): 279-84.

Chapter 11: Habits For Health

1. Motivala SJ, Tomiyama AJ, Ziegler M, Khandrika S, Irwin MR. "Nocturnal levels of ghrelin and leptin and sleep in chronic insomnia." *Psychoneuroendocrinology*. 2009 May: 34 (4): 540-545.

2. Floam S, Simpson N, Nemeth E, Scott-Sutherland J, Gautam S, Haack M. "Sleep characteristics as predictor variables of stress systems markers in insomnia disorder." *J Sleep Res*. 2014 Dec 18.

3. "Take a deep breath." Harvard Health Publications Harvard Medical School, May 2009. Retrieved September 22, 2014.

4. Tomičić M, Petric D, Rumboldt M, Carevi V, Rumboldt Z. "Deep breathing: A simple test for white coat effect detection in primary care." *Blood Press*. 2015 Jun; 24(3):158-63.

5. van der Ploeg HP, Chey T, Korda RJ, Banks E, Bauman A. "Sitting time and all-cause mortality risk in 222, 497 Australian adults". "*Arch Intern Med*. 2012; 172 (6):

6. van der Ploeg HP, Chey T, Korda RJ, Banks E, Bauman A. "Sitting time and all-cause mortality risk in 222, 497 Australian adults". "*Arch Intern Med*. 2012; 172 (6):

7. Kapil U, Bhadoria AS. "Television viewing and overweight and obesity amongst children." *Biomed J.* 2014 Aug 28.

8. "Regular exercise plays a consistent and significant role in reducing fatigue." *Science Daily*, 8 November 2006. Retrieved September 2014.

9. "Talking of walking in three easy pieces." *Harvard Health Letter*, March 2011. Retrieved September 2014.

10. Carek PJ, Laibstain SE, Carek SM. "Exercise for the treatment of depression and anxiety." *Int J Psychiatry Med.* 2011;41(1):15-28.

11. Legrand FD. "Effects of exercise on physical self-concept, global self-esteem, and depression in women of low socioeconomic status with elevated depressive symptoms." *J Sport Exerc Psychol.* 2014 Aug; 36(4): 357-65.

Chapter 12: Healthy Eating On The Go

1. Mahan LK, Escott-Stump S. *Krause's Food, Nutrition, and Diet Therapy.* 11th edition. Elsevier, 2004.

2. "Healthy fast food. Tips for making healthier fast food choices." *Helpguide.org.* nd. Retrieved September 29, 2014.

3. Sánchez-Villegas A, Toledo E, de Irala J, Ruiz-Canela M, Pla-Vidal J, Martínez-González MA. "Fast-food and commercial baked goods consumption and the risk of depression. *Public Health Nutr.* 2012 Mar: 15(3): 424-32.

4. Rohrmann S, Overvad K, Bueno-de-Mesquita HB, et al. "Meat consumption and mortality—results from the European Prospective Investigation into Cancer and Nutrition." *BMC Med.* 2013;11:63

5. Kaluza J, Akesson A, Wolk A. "Processed and unprocessed red meat consumption and risk of heart failure: prospective study of men." *Circ Heart Fail.* 2014;7:552-557.

6. Hone-Blanchet A, Fecteau S. "Overlap of food addiction and substance use disorders definitions: analysis of animal and human studies." *Neuropharmacology.* 2014 Oct; 85: 81-90.

7. Rao, Goutham. "Office-based strategies for the management of obesity." *American Family Physician.* 2010 June 15; 81(12): 1449-1455.

Chapter 13: Nutritious Lunches And Snacks

1. M. Hendy H. "Effectiveness of trained peer models to encourage food acceptance in preschool children." *Appetite.* 2002; 39(3): 217–225

2. Young EM, Fors SW, Hayes DM. "Associations between perceived parent behaviors and middle school student fruit and vegetable consumption." *Journal of Nutrition Education Behavior.* 2004; 36(1):2–8

3. Cullen KW, Baranowski T, Rittenberry L, Cosart C, Hebert D, de Moor C. "Child-reported family and peer influences on fruit, juice and vegetable consumption: reliability and validity of measures." *Health Education Research.* 2001;16 (2):187–200.

4. Rhee KE, Lumeng JC, Appugliese DP, Kaciroti N, Bradley RH. "Parenting styles and overweight status in first grade." *Pediatrics.* 2006; 117(6): 2047–2054.

5. Birch LL, Birch D, Marlin DW, Kramer L. "Effects of instrumental consumption on children's food preference." *Appetite.* 1982; 3(2):125–134.

6. Birch L, Marlin D, Rotter J. "Eating as the means activity in a contingency: effects on young children's food preference". *Child Development*. 1984; 55:432–439.

7. Birch L, McPhee L, Shoba BC, Steinberg L, Krehbiel R. "Clean up your plate: effects of child feeding practices on the conditioning of meal size." *Learning and motivation*. 1987;18: 301–317.

8. Mischel W, Shoda Y, Rodriguez MI. "Delay of gratification in children." *Science*. 1989; 244(4907):933–938.

9. Mischel W, Shoda Y, Rodriguez MI. "Delay of gratification in children." *Science*. 1989; 244(4907):933–938.

10. Carruth BR, Ziegler P, Gordon A, Barr SI. "Prevalence of picky eaters among infants and toddlers and their caregiver's decisions about offering a food." *Journal of the American Dietetic Association*. 2004; 104:S57–S64.

11. Birch LL, Marlin DW. "I don't like it; I never tried it: effects of exposure on two-year-old children's food preferences." *Appetite*. 1982; 3: 353–360.

Chapter 14: Shopping Guide And Everyday Superfoods

1. Cho YS, Baik SH, Park HS, Rhu NS, Cho DI, Kim JW. "Clinical features of sulfite-sensitive asthmatics." *Tuberc Respir Dis*. 1992;39:159–166.

2. Di Lorenzo G, Pacor ML, Mansueto P, Martinelli N, Esposito-Pellitteri M, Lo Bianco C, et al. "Food-additive-induced urticaria: a survey of 838 patients with recurrent chronic idiopathic urticaria." *Int Arch Allergy Immunol*. 2005;138:235–242.

3. García-Gavín J, Parente J, Goossens A. "Allergic contact dermatitis caused by sodium metabisulfite: a challenging allergen: a case series and literature review." *Contact Dermatitis*. 2012;67:260–269.

4. Schwartz HJ. "Sensitivity to ingested metabisulfite: variations in clinical presentation." *J Allergy Clin Immunol*. 1983;71:487–489.

5. Vally H, Misso NL, Madan V. "Clinical effects of sulphite additives." *Clin Exp Allergy*. 2009;39:1643–1651.

6. Jiang Y, Wu SH, Shu XO, Xiang YB, Ji BT, Milne GL, Cai Q, Zhang X, Gao YT, Zheng W, Yang G. "Cruciferous vegetable intake is inversely correlated with circulating levels of proinflammatory markers in women." *J Acad Nutr Diet*. 2014 May;114(5):700-8.e2.

7. "Eating cruciferous vegetables may improve breast cancer survival." Vanderbilt University Medical Center. 3 April, 2012. Web. 29 Sept, 2014.

8. Verhoeven DT, Goldbohm RA, van Poppel G, Verhagen H, van den Brandt PA. "Epidemiological studies on brassica vegetables and cancer risk." *Cancer Epidemiology, Biomarkers and Prevention*. 1996 Sept; Vol 5, 733-748.

9. Xiong XJ, Wang PQ, Li SJ, Li XK, Zhang YQ, Wang J. "Garlic for hypertension: A systematic review and meta-analysis of randomized controlled trials." *Phytomedicine*. 2015 Mar 15;22(3):352-61.

10. Arreola R, Quintero-Fabián S, López-Roa RI, Flores-Gutiérrez EO, Reyes-Grajeda JP, Carrera-Quintanar L, Ortuño-Sahagún D. "Immunomodulation and anti-inflammatory effects of garlic compounds." *J Immunol Res*. 2015;2015:401630.

11. Ravn-Haren G, Dragsted LO, Buch-Andersen T, Jensen EN, Jensen RI, Németh-Balogh M, Paulovicsová B, Bergström A, Wilcks A, Licht TR, Markowski J, Bügel S. "Intake of whole apples or clear apple juice has contrasting effects on plasma lipids in healthy volunteers." *Eur J Nutr*. 2013 Dec;52(8):1875-89.

12. Hebeisen DF, Hoeflin F, Reusch HP, Junker E, Lauterburg BH. "Increased concentrations of omega-3 fatty acids in milk and platelet rich plasma of grass-fed cows." *Int J Vitam Nutr Res.* 1993;63(3):229-33.

13. CA Daley, Abbott A, Doyle PA, Nader GA, Larson A. "A review of fatty acid profiles and antioxidant content in grass-fed and grain-fed beef." *Nutr J.* 2010 Mar 10; 9:10.

14. Marie-Pierre St-Onge and Peter J. H. Jones. "Physiological effects of medium-chain triglycerides: potential agents in the prevention of obesity." J. Nutr. 2002; 132 (3):329-332.

Recipes

1. Winham DM, Hutchins AM, Johnston CJ. "Pinto bean consumption reduces biomarkers for heart disease risk." *J Am Coll Nutr.* 2007; 26(3):243-249.

2. Othman RA, Moghadasian MH, Jones PJ. "Cholesterol-lowering effects of oat β-glucan." *Nutr Rev.* 2011 Jun; 69(6):299-309.

3. Keegan RJ, Lu Z, Bogusz JM, Williams JE, Holick MF. "Photobiology of vitamin D in mushrooms and its bioavailability in humans." *Dermatoendocrinol.* 2013 Jan 1; 5(1):165-76.

4. Gunawardena D, Bennett L, Shanmugam K, King K, Williams R, Zabaras D, Head R, Ooi L, Gyengesi E, Münch G. "Anti-inflammatory effects of five commercially available mushroom species determined in lipopolysaccharide and interferon-γ activated murine macrophages." *Food Chem.* 2014 Apr 1; 148: 92-6.

5. Fernandex, ML. "Dietary cholesterol provided by eggs and plasma lipoproteins in healthy populations." *Curr Opin Clin Nutr Metab Care.* 2006 Jan; 9 (1): 8-12.

6. Karr JE, Alexander JE, Winningham RG. "Omega-3 polyunsaturated fatty acids and cognition throughout the lifespan: a review." *Nutr Neurosci.* 2011 Sep; 14(5):216-25.

7. Saremi A, Arora R. "The utility of omega-3 fatty acids in cardiovascular disease." *Am J Ther.* 2009 Sep-Oct; 16 (5):421-36.

8. Easton MD, Luszniak D, Von der GE. "Preliminary examination of contaminant loadings in farmed salmon, wild salmon and commercial salmon feed." *Chemosphere.* 2002 Feb; 46 (7):1053-74.

9. Jenkins DJ, Mirrahimi A, Srichaikul K, Berryman CE, Wang L, Carleton A, Abdulnour S, Sievenpiper JL, Kendall CW, Kris-Etherton PM. "Soy protein reduces serum cholesterol by both intrinsic and food displacement mechanisms." *J Nutr.* 2010 Dec; 140 (12): 2302S-2311S.

10. van Poppel G, Verhoeven DT, Verhagen H, Goldbohm RA. "Brassica vegetables and cancer prevention. Epidemiology and mechanisms." *Adv Exp Med Biol.* 1999; 472: 159-68.

11. Jenkins D, Kendall C, Josse A, et al. "Almonds decrease post-prandial glycemia, insulinemia, and oxidative damage in healthy individuals." *J Nutr.* 2006; 136: 2987–92.

Index

ABOUT THE AUTHORS

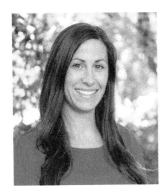

Dr. Julie Briley is a naturopathic physician, educator, and mother. She is the co-founder of the Food As Medicine Institute at National College of Natural Medicine in Portland, Oregon, and a faculty member in the Master of Science in Nutrition program.

At her private practice in downtown Portland, Dr. Briley focuses on identifying food sensitivities, optimizing digestive health, balancing hormones, and the prevention and treatment of chronic diseases. She is a popular speaker in Portland's thriving health and food culture.

Dr. Briley's longstanding interest in community health and education was sparked through her research and teaching experience in the U.S and Latin America, including her service as a Peace Corps volunteer in Paraguay.

Dr. Briley received her doctorate degree at National College of Natural Medicine and her Bachelors of Science in Biology from University of Wisconsin at Madison.

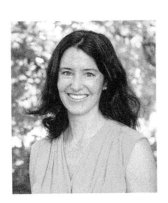

Dr. Courtney Jackson is a naturopathic physician who passionately promotes the healing power of whole foods to her patients and the public. She is the creator of the ECO Project at the National College of Natural Medicine and co-founder of the Food as Medicine Institute.

Prior to pursuing her medical career, Dr. Jackson earned her Bachelor of Science in Resource Ecology Management from the University of Michigan. Her interest in medicine stemmed from growing up in a conventional medical family in the Midwest. Her ND degree beautifully rounds out the medical family tree and adds a dynamic flavor to family conversations.

Dr. Jackson maintains a private practice in southeast Portland where she offers comprehensive, patient-centered evaluations focusing on hormone, digestive, and cardiovascular health. She loves spending time indoors and outdoors with her husband and two kids and celebrating a good meal with them.

ABOUT NCNM Press

NCNM Press, a division of National College of Natural Medicine, publishes distinctive titles that enrich the history, clinical practice, and growing significance of contemporary natural medicine systems. As well, the Press strives with its titles to recognize historical and contemporary best practices in environmental, global health, and sustainability research and history.

NCNM (National College of Natural Medicine, Portland, Oregon) was founded in 1956. Its program includes the longest serving accredited naturopathic program in North America and five highly regarded graduate research programs in Nutrition, Global Health, Integrative Medicine Research, and Integrative Mental Health. NCNM also offers undergraduate programs in Holistic Health Studies and in Nutrition. As well, the College is home to one of North America's most unique classical Chinese medicine programs, embracing the traditions, history, roots and lineage community so essential as a powerful mentoring model for future practitioners. Its rare book collection on natural medicine is the largest and most complete of its kind in North America.

CPSIA information can be obtained
at www.ICGtesting.com
Printed in the USA
FSOW03n0115200916
25118FS